Atlas of Surgery of the Stomach, Duodenum, and Small Bowel

The Atlases of Operative Surgery

Series Editor

R. Scott Jones, M.D.
Professor and Chairman
Department of Surgery
The University of Virginia
Charlottesville, Virginia

PUBLISHED AND FORTHCOMING VOLUMES

Daly & Cady/ATLAS OF SURGICAL ONCOLOGY

Donovan/ATLAS OF TRAUMA SURGERY

Lamberth & Doty/PERIPHERAL VASCULAR SURGERY

Jones/ATLAS OF LIVER AND BILIARY SURGERY

Kaiser/ATLAS OF GENERAL THORACIC SURGERY

Ponsky/ATLAS OF SURGICAL ENDOSCOPY

Reber & Zinner/ATLAS OF PANCREATIC SURGERY

Wells/ATLAS OF BREAST SURGERY

An Atlas of Operative Surgery

Atlas of Surgery of the Stomach, Duodenum, and Small Bowel

by

James C. Thompson, M.D.
John Woods Harris Professor and Chairman, Department of Surgery
University of Texas Medical Branch
Galveston, Texas

Illustrated by Lee Rose

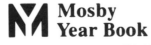

Mosby
Year Book

St. Louis   Baltimore   Boston   Chicago   London   Philadelphia   Sydney   Toronto

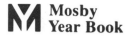

Mosby Year Book

Dedicated to Publishing Excellence

Sponsoring Editor: Nancy E. Chorpenning
Associate Managing Editor, Manuscript Services: Deborah Thorp
Production Coordinator: Nancy C. Baker
Proofroom Manager: Barbara Kelly

1 2 3 4 5 6 7 8 9 0 CL/PP 96 95 94 93 92

Library of Congress Cataloging-in-Publication Data
Thompson, James C., 1928-
    Atlas of surgery of the stomach, duodenum, and small bowel / James
C. Thompson.
        p.   cm.
    Includes bibliographical references and index.
    ISBN 0-8151-8767-X
    1. Gastrointestinal system—Surgery—Atlases. I. Title.
    [DNLM: 1. Duodenum—surgery—atlases. 2. Gastrointestinal
Diseases—surgery—atlases. 3. Intestine, Small—surgery—atlases.
    4. Stomach—surgery—atlases. WI 17 T473a]
RD540.T47 1991
617.5'53—dc20   91-22620
DNLM/DLC   CIP
for Library of Congress

*This book is dedicated with love to Patricia, Jan, Gayle, Jim, John, Laura F.,
Mike, Chris, Emily, Leah, Taylor, and Laura C.*

Series Introduction

In the 1950s and 1960s, Year Book Medical Publishers provided the surgical profession with a valuable series of books called the *Handbooks of Operative Surgery,* which were especially useful to residents. Mosby-Year Book has now introduced a new series in the same tradition—the *Atlases of Operative Surgery*—focusing on general surgery.

Certainly, diseases of the stomach, duodenum, and small intestine occupy a major portion of most general surgery practices. However, surgical treatment has changed since publication of the original handbooks by Welch *(Stomach and Duodenum)* and Greenlee *(Intestinal Surgery).* For example, frequency of stress and duodenal ulcers and gastric cancer has decreased. Yet, when present, they are often managed surgically, now with new and improved tools and techniques.

As in other disciplines, overall management of gastrointestinal disease has improved significantly in the past two decades. Our greater understanding of the natural history and pathophysiology of disease, better drugs, advanced imaging technology, and improved endoscopic techniques combine to make the safety and effectiveness of surgical management better than ever. For these reasons, the timing is perfect for a new book on surgery of the stomach, duodenum and small intestine to crystallize current thinking and technical approaches.

Surgeons in training and in practice will welcome Dr. Thompson's *Atlas of Surgery of the Stomach, Duodenum, and Small Bowel.* This excellent volume provides comprehensive and detailed attention to every aspect of surgical management of gastroduodenal and intestinal disease. Dr. Thompson's extensive experience and his mastery of writing have produced a text of unparalleled logic, clarity, and precision. In addition, this book is a pleasure to read. The even and fluid style, the well-chosen expression of personal preferences, and the effective and timely inclusion of anecdotes enliven the text and convey a feeling of private lessons from a master surgeon and a master teacher.

Dr. Thompson has practiced gastrointestinal surgery for more than 35 years and possesses keen judgment and technical skills. In addition, his remarkable record of scientific productivity and accomplishment have earned for him the surgical world's highest respect as a surgical scientist-clinician. That background of clinical knowledge and skill, scientific discipline, and superior writing skill have produced a text on the craft of surgery written with a critical and a balanced view. Experienced surgeons, residents, and students all will enjoy reading Dr. Thompson's *Atlas of Surgery of the Stomach, Duodenum, and Small Bowel.* In addition to the enjoyment they will learn many new things, as I did.

R. Scott Jones, M.D.
S. Hurt Watts Professor and Chairman
Department of Surgery
University of Virginia Health Sciences Center
Charlottesville, Virginia

Preface

First, I would like to acknowledge the outstanding former editions of *Surgery of the Stomach and Duodenum* by Claude Welch, published by Year Book Medical Publishers, 1951 to 1966. Those volumes were of great help to me in my residency and later training, and I hope this book will provide similar help to others.

Anyone with vision can foresee within the next decade many small revolutions in adaptations of minimally invasive surgical techniques (via laparoscopy) to manage abdominal pathologic lesions. This atlas summarizes the way we operate on patients with pathologic lesions of the stomach, duodenum, or small bowel, nine years before the end of this century.

The general format in each of the three major sections of this atlas (stomach, duodenum, and small bowel) is to discuss and depict anatomy and blood supply, to provide a discussion of diagnostic studies where indicated, to cover management of congenital lesions, and then to cover operative procedures for common pathologic lesions.

In the stomach section, we arbitrarily included discussion of Nissen fundoplication for reflux esophagitis caused by hiatal hernia. In a similar vein, since peptic ulcer disease is shared by the stomach and duodenum, we have included all operative procedures for duodenal ulcer in the section on the stomach (even those procedures performed on the duodenum itself).

In the duodenum section the reader will find discussion and depiction of radical pancreaticoduodenectomy (Whipple procedure) in the management of cancer of the papilla of Vater or of the duodenum itself.

Mechanical obstruction is one of the most common indications for operation on the small bowel. We have included under mechanical obstruction discussion only of adhesions, intussusception, and gallstone ileus. Other pathologic lesions that may or may not cause bowel obstruction (hernias, tumors, and Crohn's disease) are discussed separately. At the end of the small bowel section we present a section on techniques, in which we arbitrarily include discussion of drainage of pancreatic pseudocysts, either cystgastrostomy or Roux-en-Y cystjejunostomy.

Further information on diseases of the stomach and duodenum is provided in a chapter that I wrote (Sabiston DC: *Textbook of Surgery,* ed 14. Philadelphia, WB Saunders, 1991, and further information on the small bowel may be found in a chapter that I wrote with co-author Courtney Townsend (Schwartz SI: *Principles of Surgery,* ed 5. New York, McGraw-Hill, 1989).

James C. Thompson, M.D.

Acknowledgments

I would like to express gratitude to all those who have helped with the preparation of this book. The splendid artist, Lee Rose, has provided the magnificent illustrations that clarify all segments of this book. I had a great deal of fun working with him and it was an immense privilege to have such an innovative colleague. Dr. William H. Nealon, chief of our endoscopy service, provided wise advice and counsel. I want to thank Drs. Charles Fagan and Leonard Swischuk of our department of radiology for their unflagging help in providing access to appropriate images (radiographs and ultrasonograms). I am greatly indebted to nurses in the operating room, particularly to Mss. Dossie Gray and Birdell Hall, and Jack LeClair, R.N. Surgical residents in our training program have been stimulating and unfailingly helpful and I would like particularly to express my appreciation to Ahmed Abdullah, M.D., Michael S. Bouton, M.D., Robert A. Campbell, M.D., Kelly R. Kunkle, M.D., Paul K. Minifee, M.D., and Louis L. Strock, M.D. Our departmental administrator, Mr. Peter Lee, has the great knack of making all large problems seem small, and I would like to express my thanks to the talented manuscript typists, Mary Lou Mraz and Grant Fairchild. I am especially indebted to my outstanding secretary, Dorothy LeFevers. My relations with Mosby-Year Book, Inc. have been particularly cordial and I am delighted with the help and encouragement provided by Ms. Nancy Chorpenning.

James C. Thompson, M.D.

Contents

STOMACH

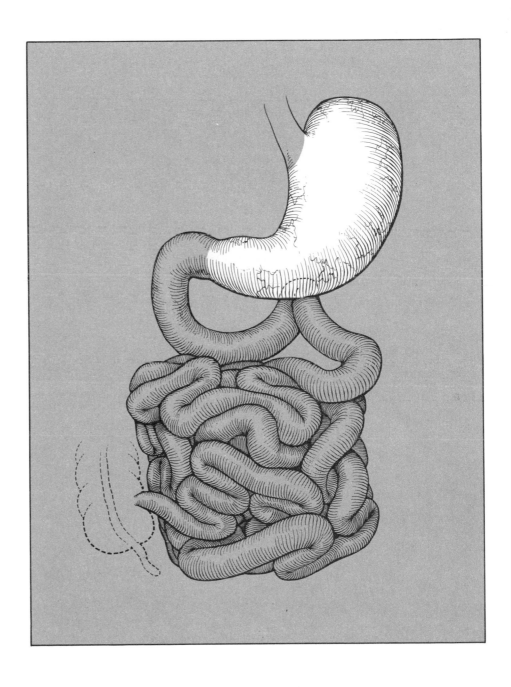

Part I

Anatomy of the Stomach

1

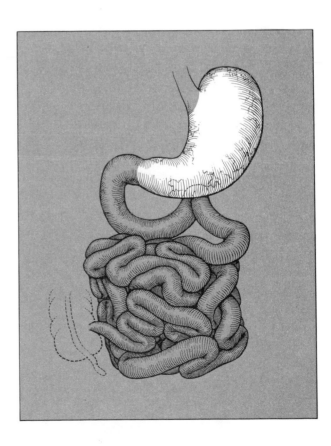

The stomach arises as a spindle-shaped dilatation of the foregut during the fourth week of embryonic life. During a later growth spurt, the stomach undergoes rotation so that the former left side of the stomach becomes the anterior wall and the former right side comes to lie posteriorly (the mnemonic for this is LARP). The duodenum, initially suspended between dorsal and ventral mesenteries, also rotates so that the second part of the duodenum becomes retroperitoneal and the first three portions encompass the head of the pancreas in the C-loop.

FIG 1–1

A. The fully developed stomach lies between the esophagus and the duodenum and is the largest dilatation of the gut. The topographic anatomy of the stomach is quite simple, although it has been made confusing by the application of overlapping terms by anatomists, surgeons, endoscopists, and radiologists. For gross description, the stomach can be divided into fundus, body, and antrum. In this schema the fundus is the dome of the stomach, to the left of and superior to the esophagogastric junction. The antrum distally has no clear external landmarks for its proximal margin, but the antrofundic border can be estimated. An angulation on the lesser curvature at about the midline of the body, about 5 to 7 cm proximal to the pylorus on the lesser curvature, is called the *incisura angularis* (shown as point *a* on the lesser curvature). The antrum is distal to a line drawn from the incisura across to the greater curvature of the stomach (in approximately the position of a line from *a* to *a'*). The so-called body of the stomach is between the fundus and antrum. At the gastroduodenal junction, the pylorus can be palpated as a thick ring of muscle; it is marked externally by the prominent veins of Mayo in the anterior serosa. These veins (see **C**, p 7) mark the boundary between the stomach and duodenum. Functional studies on the stomach have shown it to consist of only two functional areas, the fundus (or oxyntic gland area) and the antrum (pyloric gland area). The mucosa of the fundus secretes acid-peptic juice and histologically is seen to have deep gastric glands that contain mucous cells, epithelial cells, chief cells, which secrete pepsinogen, parietal cells, which secrete acid, and argentaffin cells, whose function is not entirely understood. Some of these cells seem to contain somatostatin; others may have vasoactive intestinal peptide. There are, additionally, mast cells in the mucosa whose cytoplasmic granules contain multiple substances, prominent among which is histamine. The exocrine secretion of the fundus is acid-peptic juice, whereas the antrum secretes a thick, viscid, relatively alkaline mucus. The antral mucosa, of course, also contains specialized endocrine cells that elaborate gastrin and somatostatin. Again, the division between the functional area of the fundus and antrum is on a line drawn from *a* to *a'*. Some general landmarks will be given, but it should be noted that they are subject to great individual variations; some persons have a horizontally placed stomach, others have a long, vertical J-shaped organ. The esophagogastric junction, called the cardia, is located just to the left of the tenth thoracic vertebra, and the gastroduodenal junction, the pylorus, is located just to the right of the midline at about the interspace between the first and second lumbar vertebrae. The superior margin of the stomach between the cardia and the pylorus (a distance of about 12 to 14 cm) is the lesser curvature of the stomach, suspended from the liver by the gastrohepatic ligament, which in turn forms the superior portion of the anterior wall of the lesser omental bursa. The inferolateral convex border of the stomach is the greater curvature, which is nearly three times as long as the lesser curvature. From the major portion of the greater curvature is suspended the gastrocolic ligament connecting the greater curvature of the stomach with the superior margin of the transverse colon. The gastrocolic ligament forms the lower portion of the anterior wall of the lesser omental bursa, of which the midportion is the posterior wall of the stomach itself.

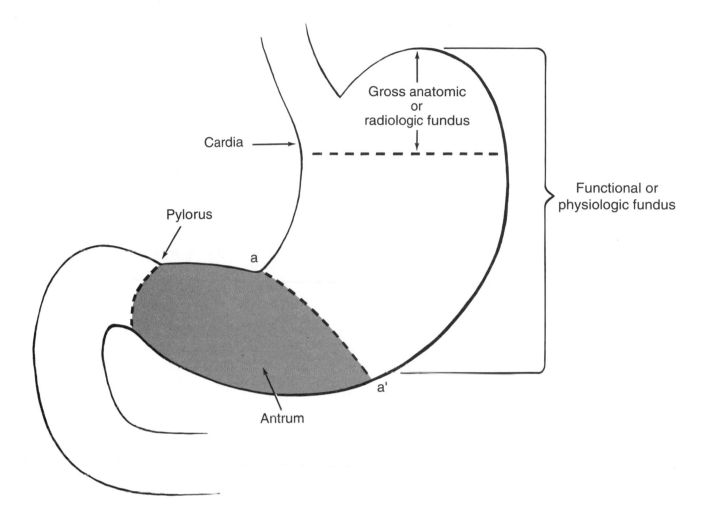

B. The arterial supply of the stomach is particularly rich. The arrangement of the individual vessels shows innumerable variations and the schema shown here is only one of many. In most persons, six vessels provide the main blood supply; these are the left and right gastric arteries, which supply the area of the lesser curvature; the left and right gastroepiploic arteries, which supply the greater curvature; the splenic artery, which supplies the area of the fundus by way of the short gastric arteries; and the gastroduodenal artery, which sends branches to the area of the pylorus. The gastroepiploic arch is usually complete, so that the entire greater curvature can almost always be maintained by either the right or left gastroepiploic artery. A rich anastomotic network is evident, and no area is served by end-arteries. N.A. Michaels (*Blood Supply of Upper Abdominal Organs*. Philadelphia, JB Lippincott, 1955, p 248) made a meticulous study of the blood supply of the stomach and called attention to possible surgical hazards (for example, in more than 20% of people the primary or secondary blood supply of the left lobe of the liver would be lost if the left gastric artery were divided at its origin). Several other arteries are worthy of note. In doing a very high gastric resection for cancer, if the left gastric and splenic arteries are divided, the proximal stomach may be supplied by descending esophageal branches from the left inferior phrenic artery. A posterior eroding duodenal ulcer, usually located in the superior margin of the bulb, may frequently erode directly into the main gastroduodenal artery itself, producing massive blood loss. In ligating the base of a bleeding duodenal ulcer, it is well to remember that bleeding may persist owing to anastomotic connections from the transverse pancreatic artery. Berne and Rosoff have advocated separate ligation of this vessel by means of the so-called U stitch (see Chapter 17).

C. This figure shows the venous drainage of the stomach. The veins in general follow the distribution of the arteries except that the veins of the lesser curvature (coronary vein on the left and right gastric or pyloric vein on the right) drain directly into the portal vein. The coronary vein may be ligated or anastomosed to the inferior vena cava in operations for bleeding esophageal varices. The right gastric and pancreaticoduodenal veins drain into the superior mesenteric vein and the left gastroepiploic and short gastric veins drain into the splenic vein.

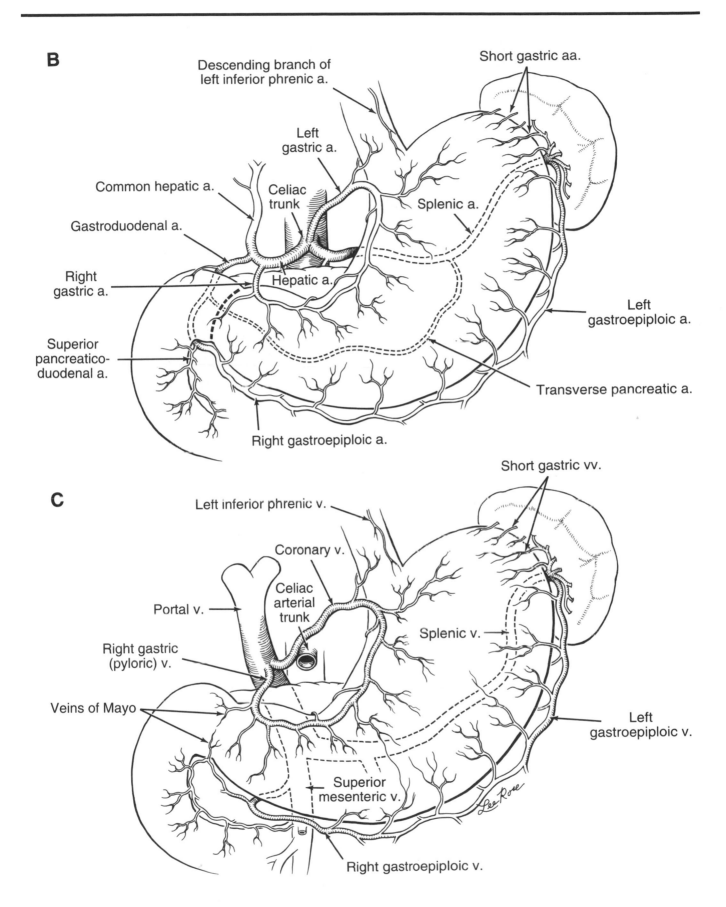

B

Short gastric aa.

Descending branch of
left inferior phrenic a.

Left
gastric a.

Common hepatic a.

Celiac
trunk

Gastroduodenal a.

Splenic a.

Right
gastric a.

Hepatic a.

Left
gastroepiploic a.

Superior
pancreatico-
duodenal a.

Transverse pancreatic a.

Right gastroepiploic a.

C

Short gastric vv.

Left inferior phrenic v.

Coronary v.

Portal v.

Celiac
arterial
trunk

Right gastric
(pyloric) v.

Splenic v.

Veins of Mayo

Left
gastroepiploic v.

Superior
mesenteric v.

Right gastroepiploic v.

D. This depicts the anatomy of the vagi. The vagal nerves in the upper posterior mediastinum begin to decussate about the esophagus at a point near the inferior margin of the aortic arch, from which point the left and right vagi intermingle freely. In the midthorax, some of these vagal fibers enter the muscular wall of the esophagus and traverse the entire distal thorax and upper abdomen, embedded within the muscle wall. For this reason, it is often impossible to completely divide all vagal fibers unless the esophagus is transected. Usually the vagi coalesce just above the diaphragm into a small left (anterior) vagal trunk and a right (or posterior) vagal trunk that is almost twice as large. The posterior trunk sends a branch to the celiac ganglia and the left or anterior trunk sends a branch to the liver and gallbladder. Both nerves have numerous small esophageal branches and usually a fairly large fundic branch (one of which, in dissection for selective proximal vagotomy, is often found near the angle of His, as the so-called criminal nerve of Grassi). The remainder of the anterior and posterior vagi then descend inferiorly along the lesser curvature as the nerves of Latarjet, running in the lower margin of the gastrohepatic ligament, near the point where the ligament attaches to the stomach. The nerves of Latarjet give off numerous branches to the acid-secreting fundus and then cross onto the lesser curvature in an arrangement frequently referred to as a crow's foot. The antral branches of the vagi provide motor innervation to the circular smooth muscle of the antrum, which is the pump that empties the stomach. Truncal vagotomy therefore denervates the antrum and converts the stomach into a flaccid sac. Selective proximal vagotomy (also called, among other terms, parietal cell vagotomy, selective gastric vagotomy, proximal gastric vagotomy, and supraselective vagotomy) severs the vagal branches to the acid-secreting fundus but preserves the motor branches to the antrum, thereby achieving the long-sought physiologic goal of reducing acidity without the necessity of a drainage procedure. Controversy has arisen regarding the extent of proximal and distal denervation of the stomach in selective proximal vagotomy procedures. Most authorities now agree that the denervation of the proximal stomach and esophagus should be carried all the way to the esophageal hiatus of the diaphragm. The problem is how far distal denervation should be carried. Excessive denervation interferes with gastric emptying, but failure to take distal nerves that pass in retrograde to the fundus may yield persistent high acid output. We choose an arbitrary point on the lesser curvature 7 cm proximal to the pylorus and inspect the crow's foot at this point; any fibers ranging proximally are divided.

E. The lymphatic drainage of the stomach follows the veins. Operations for malignancy of the stomach should remove as many local and regional lymph nodes as possible. For this reason, the entire gastrocolic ligament is excised, as is the gastrohepatic ligament. In the latter dissection, care should be taken to remove as many of the left gastric, celiac, and portal lymph nodes as possible. Posterior to the stomach, a chain of lymphatics follows the splenic vein, the superior mesenteric vein, and the pancreaticoduodenal and gastroduodenal veins. The submucosal lymphatic network is particularly rich in the stomach and spread of malignant cells from relatively small mucosal foci to regional lymph nodes often occurs quite early. Wangensteen at one time advocated splenectomy for any gastric cancer with the idea of removing the nodes in the splenic hilum, but that advice, along with his suggestion that the tail of the pancreas might also be taken routinely, has not been borne out by improved survival rates in operations for gastric cancer. It should be mentioned that the formal operative protocol devised by the Japanese Cancer Society stipulates dissection of the celiac, portal, left gastric, and paracardial lymph nodes, in addition to routine removal of the greater and lesser omentum.

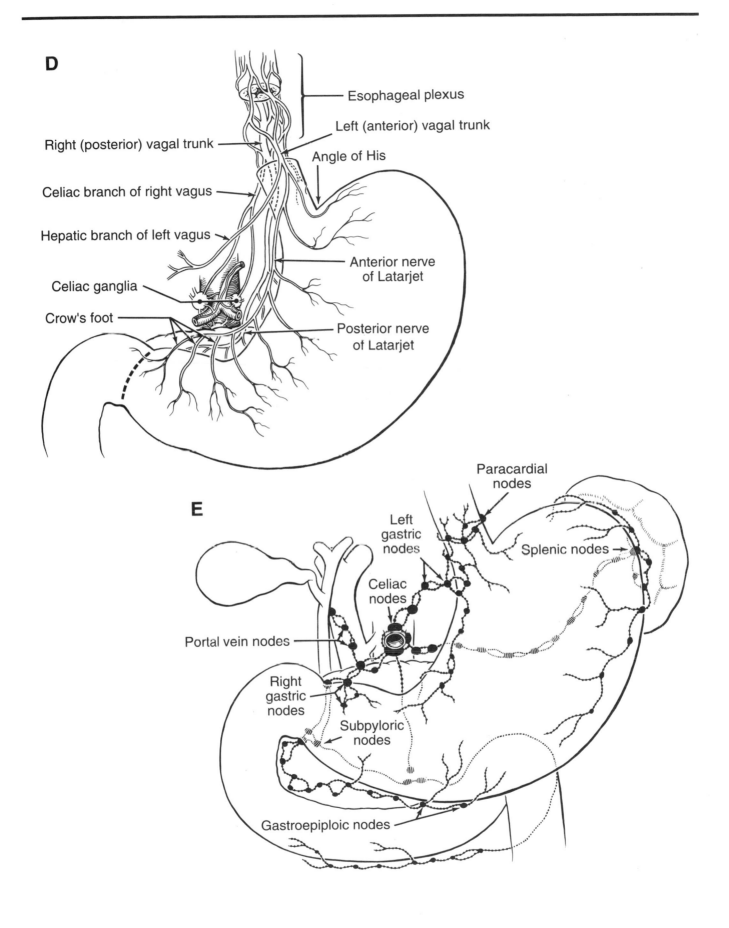

D

Esophageal plexus

Left (anterior) vagal trunk

Right (posterior) vagal trunk

Angle of His

Celiac branch of right vagus

Hepatic branch of left vagus

Celiac ganglia

Crow's foot

Anterior nerve of Latarjet

Posterior nerve of Latarjet

E

Paracardial nodes

Left gastric nodes

Splenic nodes

Celiac nodes

Portal vein nodes

Right gastric nodes

Subpyloric nodes

Gastroepiploic nodes

Diagnostic Endoscopy

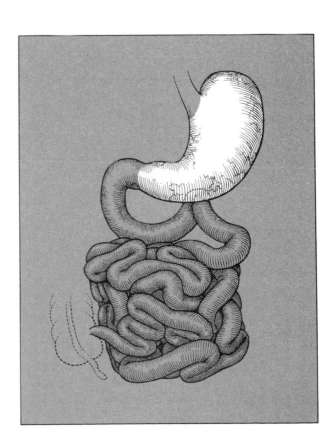

2

As recently as two decades ago, the standard diagnostic study for the proximal gut was a barium x-ray study. Now, the great advantage of endoscopy in every area of comparison (except for cost and patient discomfort) is apparent to all. Were it not for the cost, endoscopy would almost certainly replace upper gastrointestinal x-ray studies, impelled by greater accuracy (routine diagnosis of a bulbar ulcer of the duodenum is 70% accurate by x-ray and 90% to 95% accurate by endoscopy) and by the additional dynamic clinical information provided. For example, a patient with upper GI bleeding might have a duodenal or gastric ulcer, varices, gastritis, or a Mallory-Weiss tear. Endoscopy could anatomically locate all five lesions (vs. three for radiology); in addition endoscopy would show whether the anatomic lesion was bleeding. Because of this superiority and because many surgeons perform endoscopy, discussion here will be limited to endoscopy, although all surgeons depend heavily on classic GI radiology, visceral angiography, ultrasound, magnetic resonance imaging, and especially computed tomography. Routine availability of fiberoptic endoscopy has tremendously facilitated diagnosis of upper gastrointestinal lesions. Proper application of these techniques has minimized or evaporated many vexing problems: Is this gastric ulcer benign or malignant? What is the site of hemorrhage in this alcoholic patient? In this narrowed, scarred duodenum, can the pediatric (that is, small) scope pass the zone of contraction? Why is this patient jaundiced? Could he or she have a tumor or diverticulum at the duodenal papilla? Will removal of this foreign body require operation, or can it be extracted endoscopically? Will bleeding from this duodenal ulcer be likely to require operation? Is the patient's hematemesis the result of an ulcer, or a varix, or gastritis, and, if gastritis, what is the extent of the involvement? Although several controlled studies have failed to show that early endoscopy has brought about any decrease in mortality in patients with massive upper GI hemorrhage, we and others believe that early endoscopic diagnosis of the cause of bleeding greatly facilitates proper care of the patient. To mention only one point: it is vitally important to rule in or out the possibility of variceal hemorrhage, since these patients require entirely different and specific techniques of management. All therapeutic planning is facilitated by knowing the source of bleeding. Therapeutic applications of endoscopy will be discussed separately, but these applications often allow us to treat patients without operation. Often, recurrent problems such as removal of bezoars or of swallowed metallic foreign bodies in mentally deranged patients can be managed endoscopically. This is as good a place as any to vigorously exhort all surgical training program directors to provide adequate endoscopy training for surgical residents. This training should not be designed merely to give lip-service to Board requirements. Safe, adequate practice of surgery of the gut requires familiarity with and skill in the endoscopy of the proximal and distal gut. Similarly, surgeons in training who intend to prepare themselves to manage problems of the proximal or distal gut should take care to become expert in endoscopy. No one should be put off by "turf" issues. These are always rooted in greed and will not stand up to a simple request to learn a technique so as to improve one's future ability to take care of sick people. All hortatory admonitions should be interpreted with caution. No surgeon who uses an endoscope only once a month will ever become a highly skilled endoscopic magician, and difficult problems should be referred to endoscopists with great experience. I have included here a few common diagnostic uses of endoscopy with which our residents are familiar. William H. Nealon, M.D., Chief of our Endoscopic Service, has provided great help in the preparation of this section. Any errors are mine. Upper gastrointestinal endoscopy is limited to the stomach and duodenum by the length of the scope. In patients suspected of having distal duodenal or jejunal lesions, we may often carefully cleanse and reclease one of the longer endoscopes (always solemnly referred to as the long scope), and use it. At times, we have visualized the proximal 10 to 15 cm of the jejunum (see **Fig 2–3,** p 19). We have also used scopes intraoperatively to detect occult bleeding sites. The scope is sterilized and the tip handed over into the operating field to be inserted into an enterotomy. Sometimes the endoscopist can visualize a tumor or bleeding site and sometimes passage of the lighted tip through the lumen of the bowel allows visualization of angiodysplastic vascular anomalies or tumors themselves through the thin bowel wall. Illustrations in this chapter will focus on common conditions or sites of endoscopic interest (for example, duodenal ulcer, papilla of Vater, and so forth).

FIG 2-1

A. Ninety-five percent of **duodenal ulcers** occur in the bulb and are easily visualized with an end-viewing scope. Some ulcers are small and their discovery will require great diligence.

B. The duodenal bulb is characterized by smooth surface mucosa without plicae circulares (shown in the left lower corner of this figure). Anterior duodenal ulcers may penetrate through the wall and perforate into the free peritoneal cavity. Posterior ulcers may penetrate into the bed of the pancreas and cause unremitting pain, or they may erode into the gastroduodenal artery and cause bleeding that is often massive.

C. This figure shows free hemorrhage from a posterior duodenal ulcer that has eroded into the gastroduodenal artery. Techniques for the operative management of this hemorrhage are described in Chapter 17. If endoscopists can actually see blood emerging from a vessel ("visible vessel"), the likelihood of continued or resumed intermittent hemorrhage is great and the patient is apt to require operative treatment.

Duodenal Ulcer

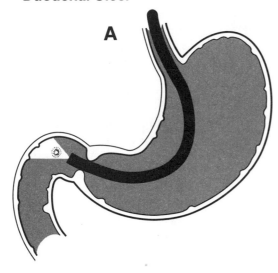

A

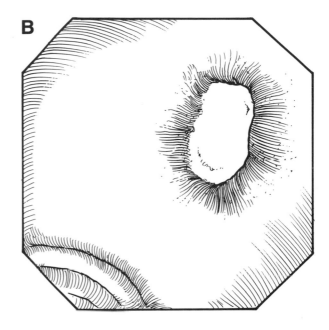

B

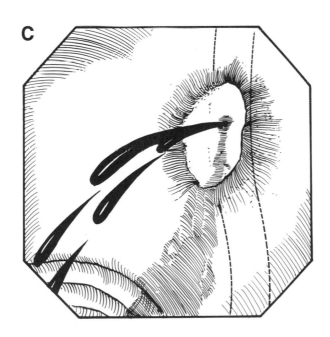

C

FIG 2–2

A. A side-viewing endoscope gives better visualization of the area of the **papilla of Vater.** For direct visualization of the papilla, this position of the tube is optimal.

B. For cannulation of the biliary tree in endoscopic retrograde cholangiography, many endoscopists extend the side-viewing scope fully along the greater curvature of the stomach. This better facilitates cannulation of the more vertical intraduodenal portion of the common bile duct, which runs parallel to the axis of the descending duodenum, just beneath the duodenal mucosa (see **D**).

C. On the other hand, cannulation of the transversely located pancreatic duct is often best achieved if the scope remains vertical along the lesser curvature and the cannula is inserted into the sphincter in an orientation that is directly perpendicular to the surface of the duodenal mucosa.

D. Viewed head-on, the papilla is often nearly hidden between folds of plicae circularis. It looks much more hemispherical than it feels at operation (where it usually feels like a small nipple). The small orifice near the center is a common channel; the bile duct is best cannulated by pointing a tube in the cephalad direction almost parallel to the surface of the duodenum, whereas the pancreatic duct is best cannulated by pointing the catheter directly perpendicular, into the orifice viewed en face, aiming at a point on the left costal margin in the midaxillary line.

E. Tumors of the papilla are often exophytic and friable. It is difficult, at times impossible, to differentiate on gross inspection between adenomas and cancer. So-called adenomas often have hidden areas of malignancy and often recur locally, and many surgeons believe that they are almost always best treated by Whipple resection (see Chapter 33).

Papilla of Vater

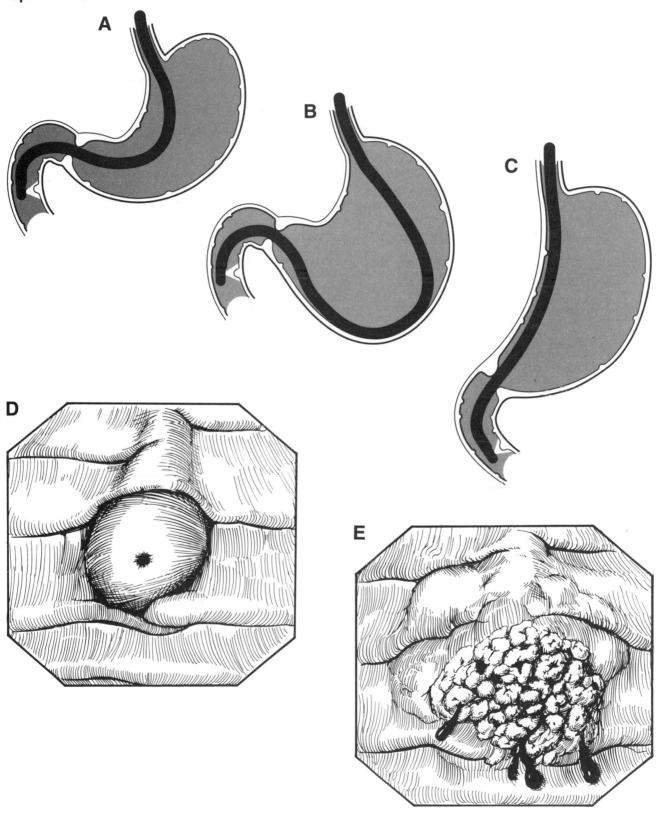

FIG 2–3

FIG 2–3

Proximal **jejunal lesions** are well within range of thoroughly cleansed longer endoscopes usually used in the distal bowel. Pathologic lesions may be visualized or (as shown here) taken by snare for biopsy.

FIG 2–4

A. **Gastritis** is a major cause of hemorrhage in alcoholics. Radiographic studies are usually of no help in diagnosing gastritis. Endoscopy can tell us not only whether the patient has gastritis, but also whether (and where) the gastritis is bleeding. This figure shows retroflexion of the gastroscope to view the area of the fundus.

B. This figure shows the *normal* retroflexed view of the proximal stomach with the endoscope coming through the gastric cardia. The vessels are prominent just beneath the mucosa.

C. By contrast, in patients with gastritis the mucosa is reddened and intensely friable, and is often bleeding briskly. Sometimes the bleeding vessels may be seen all along their course as shown here or sometimes the vessels bleed from punctate apertures. Endoscopic assessment of the extent of bleeding mucosa is important. Luminal clots impede visualization. The patient will often cooperate and vomit the clots. They are difficult to get out any other way.

Jejunal
lesions

Gastritis

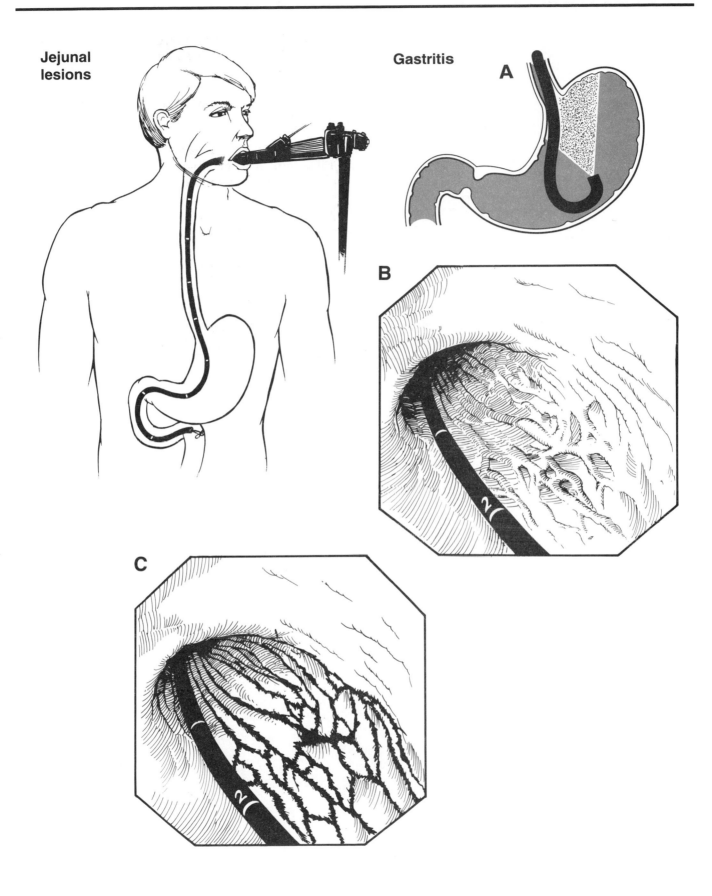

FIG 2–5

A. This figure shows visualization of distal **esophageal varices.** Again, the great advantage of endoscopy is that it can not only determine whether the patient has varices, but will indicate whether (and where) those varices are bleeding. Clearly anyone inserting a tube into the esophagus of a patient suspected of having varices should proceed with care, but we have rarely (if ever) seen damage to even the most friable varices by endoscopy. The potential is always there but with care, injury can be avoided.

B. This is a view of the distal esophagus looking into the gastric cardia. The prominent vertical folds illustrate mucosa that is bulging over varices.

C. At times, one of the varices may be covered only by an extremely thin layer of mucosa and will appear blue (the thin shading over the varix labeled *a* is intended to depict a bluish color). The mucosa over the other varices may be thicker and appear a relatively normal grayish pink.

FIG 2–6

A. Not until routine endoscopy became available for patients with upper gastrointestinal bleeding was the frequency of **tears of esophagogastric mucosa** (Mallory-Weiss syndrome) appreciated. In most series, the syndrome is responsible for 5% to 10% of major upper gastrointestinal hemorrhages. In our own large collected series reported by Villar and colleagues, 7% of patients with major upper GI hemorrhage had Mallory-Weiss tears. Preoperative diagnosis can be made only by endoscopy and such diagnosis is vital because the vast majority (99%) of these patients do not require an operation. This figure shows the retroflexed scope providing an excellent view of the tear extending from the distal esophagus into the gastric fundus. Sometimes the tears are nearly all in the esophagus, sometimes nearly all in the stomach. The frequency of prodromal vomiting varies, but it is probably more common than the 50% to 60% revealed by standard history taking. Frequently these patients are intoxicated and are poor historians.

B. The tears extend through the mucosa only and are not a prodrome to Boerhaave's syndrome of rupture of the esophagus. Bleeding usually stops spontaneously. On occasion we have used electrocoagulation to stanch a discrete bleeding point; other times we have inserted a Sengstaken-Blakemore tube, with inflation of only the gastric balloon so as to provide pressure against the bleeding mucosa. We have operated on only one patient with Mallory-Weiss syndrome in the last decade, and I am not sure that decision was correct.

Esophageal Varices

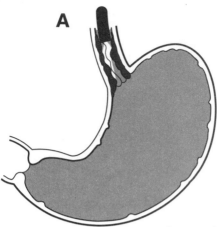

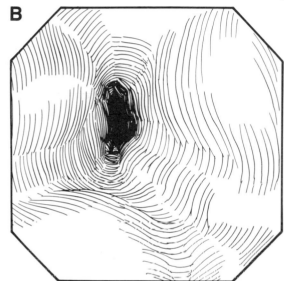

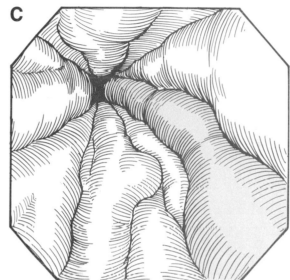

Tears of Esophagogastric Mucosa (Mallory-Weiss Syndrome)

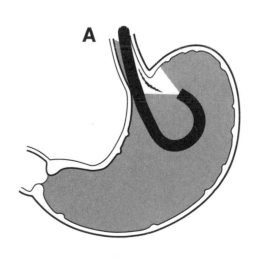

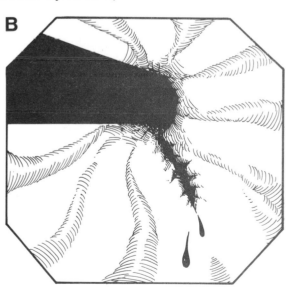

FIG 2—7

A. **Gastric polyps** may bleed, or if they protrude through the pylorus on a stalk, may cause symptoms of gastric outlet obstruction. The incidence of malignancy is not high but each polyp should be snared and retrieved for pathologic examination, taking care to note the anatomic site of the polyp.

B. Most gastric polyps are easily removed by endoscopic snare techniques. If they are on a stalk, great care should be made to include the stalk with the excised specimen. Application of electrocautery current to the snare after it is tightened around the stalk will usually ensure hemostasis. Occasionally it is necessary to touch the bleeding mucosal defect with an endoscopic cautery tip once or twice to completely stanch the bleeding.

FIG 2—8

A. Before endoscopic biopsy of **gastric ulcer** was available, one of the common indications for operation in patients with gastric ulcer was to determine whether or not the ulcer was malignant. With routine availability of endoscopic biopsy techniques, the question of whether or not an ulcer is malignant can almost always be settled prior to operation.

B. The experience of Japanese endoscopists has taught us that the accuracy of diagnosis of malignancy in gastric ulcer is greatly enhanced by taking multiple biopsies. Most articles recommend 12 separate biopsies. Eight is probably enough but it should certainly be a minimum. This shows the placement of the eight endoscopic biopsy sites. The bite of the biopsy forceps should include the rim of overhanging relatively normal mucosa where it meets the bed of the ulcer (see Chapter 7 for operative biopsy).

FIG 2—9

A. With proper use of endoscopic biopsy, it should rarely be a surprise to find **gastric cancer** in patients undergoing surgery. We routinely try to perform endoscopy on patients preoperatively; careful inspection of the stomach will almost always reveal the cancer. An exception may be patients with scirrhous carcinoma, but even in these, the abnormality of the stomach itself and the rigidity of the wall provide the clue, which can be confirmed by upper gastrointestinal radiography.

B. Cancers are usually exophytic and may often be diagnosed on the basis of gross appearance. This suspicion can be confirmed by endoscopic biopsy.

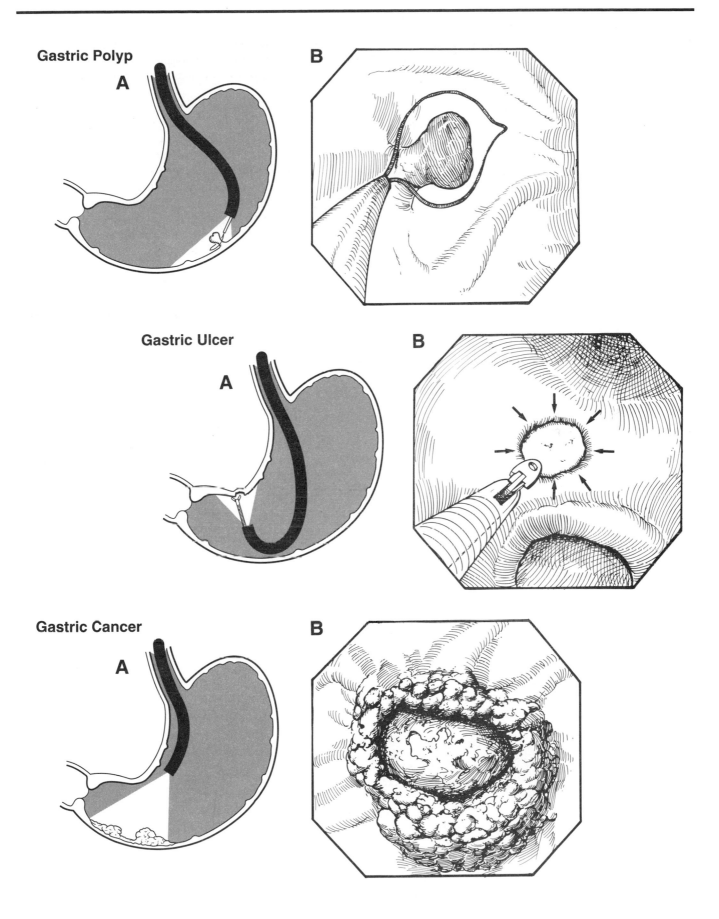

Gastric Polyp

A

B

Gastric Ulcer

A

B

Gastric Cancer

A

B

FIG 2–10

A. All scopes have one or more channels of fiberoptic bundles carrying light to the point of examination. There are other channels for other fiberoptic fibers for visualization, either for the retina or for a television camera. Other channels are available for irrigation and aspiration and passage of biopsy forceps. A small channel with a hood at the tip may be present. The purpose of the hood is to direct a stream of water (delivered through the channel) across the lens and across the tip of the scope, rather than spraying the stream of water directly away from the end of the scope. All diagnostic upper and lower endoscopes are end-viewing scopes with all the channels situated at the tip of the scope. Endoscopic retrograde cholangiopancreatography (ERCP) is performed using a side-viewing scope (shown here as JF10), in which the tip of the scope is blunt and the light source, camera, and irrigating channels are located on the side of the end of the scope. There is an open channel with a so-called bridge at the end for the purpose of manipulating the ERCP catheter into the papilla. Currently most diagnostic examinations are made with the television scope, using which the anatomy is viewed on a screen and is recorded on videotape.

B. As shown here, the endoscope can be used in varying positions in the esophagus, stomach, and duodenum to provide visualization and often tissue samples of pathologic lesions. End-viewing scopes are perhaps better for all gastric uses. The side-viewing scope is best for the duodenal papilla.

Descriptive Anatomy of the Business End of the Endoscopes

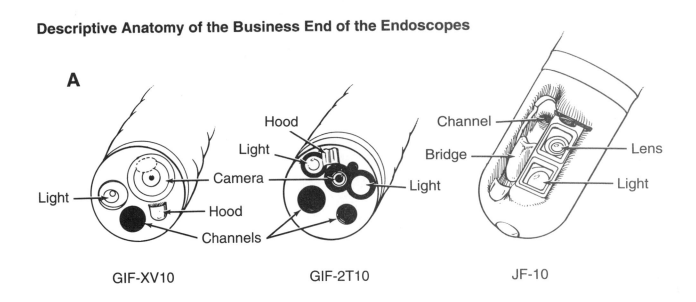

GIF-XV10   GIF-2T10   JF-10

Summary of Endoscopic Potentials

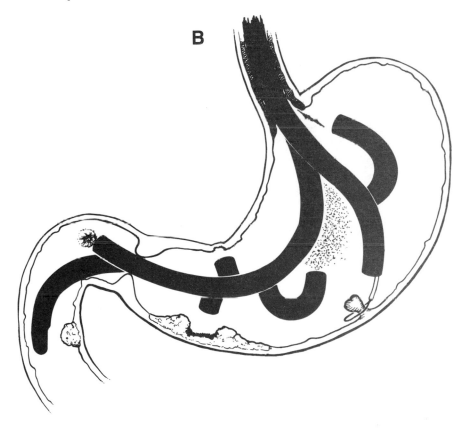

Gastric Analysis

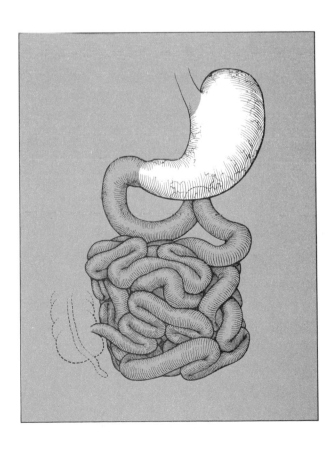

3

Twenty years ago, many gastroenterologists and gastroenteric surgeons relied heavily on measurement of acid output in an attempt to quantify the severity of an ulcer diathesis. Upper limits of normal for acid output were established for basal acid output (BAO) and maximal acid output after stimulation (MAO), for men and for women. The upper limit of BAO for women is 4 mEq/hr and for men is 6 mEq/hr; the upper limit of normal for MAO is 30 mEq/hr for women and 40 mEq/hr for men.

Carefully documented clinical studies reveal imperfect to scant correlation between acid output and clinical behavior, except in patients with the Zollinger-Ellison or other severe hypersecretory syndromes. For this reason, and because patients are not thrilled about the study, measurement of acid output has fallen into disuse except in clinical centers studying acid-peptic disease. Measurement of acid output still has clinical relevance in three situations. If a patient is suspected of having the Zollinger-Ellison syndrome, it is important to know how much acid he or she makes, since several nonulcerogenic conditions, such as pernicious anemia and chronic renal failure, give rise to hypergastrinemia; patients with Zollinger-Ellison syndrome hypersecrete both acid and gastrin. We occasionally find it worthwhile to measure acid output in patients with gastric ulcers because achlorhydria is almost always associated with a malignant ulcer. There are now better ways to diagnose malignancy preoperatively. The last indication is still important, and that is that any surgeon adopting a new acid-reducing procedure, such as selective proximal vagotomy, should measure the patient's acid output, both BAO and MAO, prior to and after operations so that the surgeon can determine whether successful reduction of acidity has been achieved by the new operative procedure. We often measure acid output in patients with distal gastric ulcers and are surprised to find out how much acid they make; in such hypersecreting persons, we may perform a truncal vagotomy as well as a distal gastric resection (although in general we believe that vagotomy is not indicated in patients with gastric ulcer).

FIG 3—1

Gastric secretion in man is measured by collecting gastric juice from fasting subjects by means of a nasogastric tube. Before insertion, the tube is measured, noting the length that will be required to enter the stomach and planning on having 15 to 20 cm of tube past the cardia. The tube is passed into the stomach and its intragastric position confirmed by instilling air and listening over the epigastrium with a stethoscope for the cavernous sound of air expelled into the stomach. Aspiration is performed and it is confirmed that gastric juice has been retrieved. Radioscopic control for placement of the tip has been recommended, but I no longer believe that it is necessary, provided that the technique described above has been used. The tube is connected to a jar to which constant suction is applied by a suction pump. Usually the first 30-minute specimen is collected and discarded, then a 30-minute sample for basal acid output is collected, and the secretory stimulant is instilled. The two stimulants now most commonly used are betazole (Histalog), 1.5 to 2.0 mg/kg, administered subcutaneously, or pentagastrin, 6 μg/kg, administered subcutaneously. The acid secretion is then collected for 2 hours in 30-minute samples. Each sample is titrated to pH 7. The results are expressed in terms of volume for a given period (usually calculated at a 1-hour equivalent) in acid concentrations (in mEq/L), and in acid output (mEq/hr). We believe that pentagastrin should be the standard stimulant since it has fewer side effects.

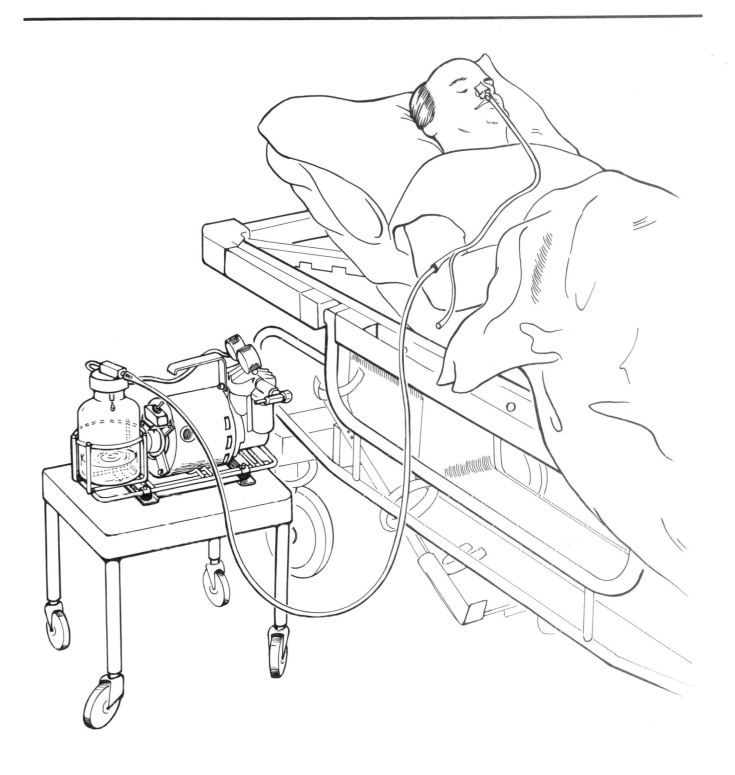

Pyloromyotomy for Congenital Hypertrophic Pyloric Stenosis

4

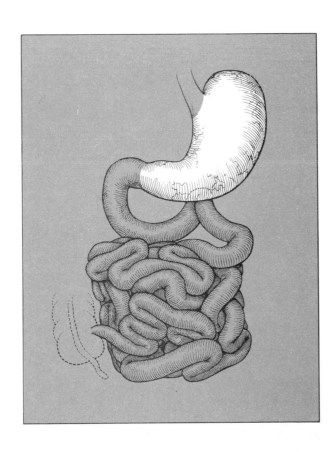

The clinical course of congenital hypertrophic pyloric stenosis is highly variable; a few children do gradually improve spontaneously and achieve complete remission without operation. Most children, however, manifest sufficient obstruction for sufficiently long periods that the operative approach is the treatment of choice. Symptoms are rarely present at birth and consist of gradually increasingly severe nonbilious vomiting. A high percentage of patients are first-born boys. Skilled pediatricians and pediatric surgeons can almost always palpate the underlying hypertrophied pylorus, the "olive." Although the diagnosis can be made clinically in the great majority of instances, it is unusual, in medical centers, for a child to undergo operation without radiologic study, although nearly everyone agrees the study is usually unnecessary. The aim at operation is to divide the hypertrophic muscle anteriorly so as to allow the underlying mucosa to pout through and relieve the obstruction. The bête noire of the procedure is accidental entry into the pyloric lumen. When this happens, the injury can usually be repaired without difficulty by means of a suture or two and by placing a tab of omentum over the pyloromyotomy. Recognition of the injury is vital.

A rare cause of congenital gastric outlet obstruction is an antral or pyloric web or diaphragm. Occasionally, these will have a small aperture so that symptoms may be delayed until late childhood or early adulthood. The diagnosis may be easily confused with pyloric stenosis in infancy and responds to simple operative excision. If the symptoms are delayed, diagnosis may be made by barium x-ray study or by endoscopy. Treatment by endoscopic electrocautery dissection may be successful, but operative removal is the usual therapy. The discussion below covers operative pyloromyotomy in infancy for congenital hypertrophic pyloric stenosis.

FIG 4–1

A. A short (2 to 3 cm) transverse incision is made in the right upper abdomen just to the right of the midline over the palpable "olive." The illustration magnifies the incision and pylorus for ease of portrayal. This shows the transverse incision and the underlying hypertrophied pylorus and proximal duodenum.

B. This cross section illustrates the thickened pyloric muscle. The dotted line indicates the zone of muscle to be divided; clearly illustrated is the danger point at which the duodenal mucosa approaches the hypertrophied pylorus, the site at which accidental injury to the mucosa most frequently occurs.

C. The pyloric "olive" is grasped with the thumb and forefinger and the pyloric muscle incised transversely. The incision is carried only partway through the muscle.

D. The pyloromyotomy is spread open with a Benson spreader, making sure that the submucosa is free of all muscle fibers and that it pouts into the wound.

E. These cross sections shows the relief of obstruction of the pylorus that is obtained with a properly performed pyloromyotomy. Again, should perforation of the mucosa occur at any point, the opening should be closed with interrupted fine sutures and the closure reinforced with omentum after a complete pyloromyotomy has been performed. Great care should be exercised to be certain that in closing the diameter of the outlet has not been narrowed.

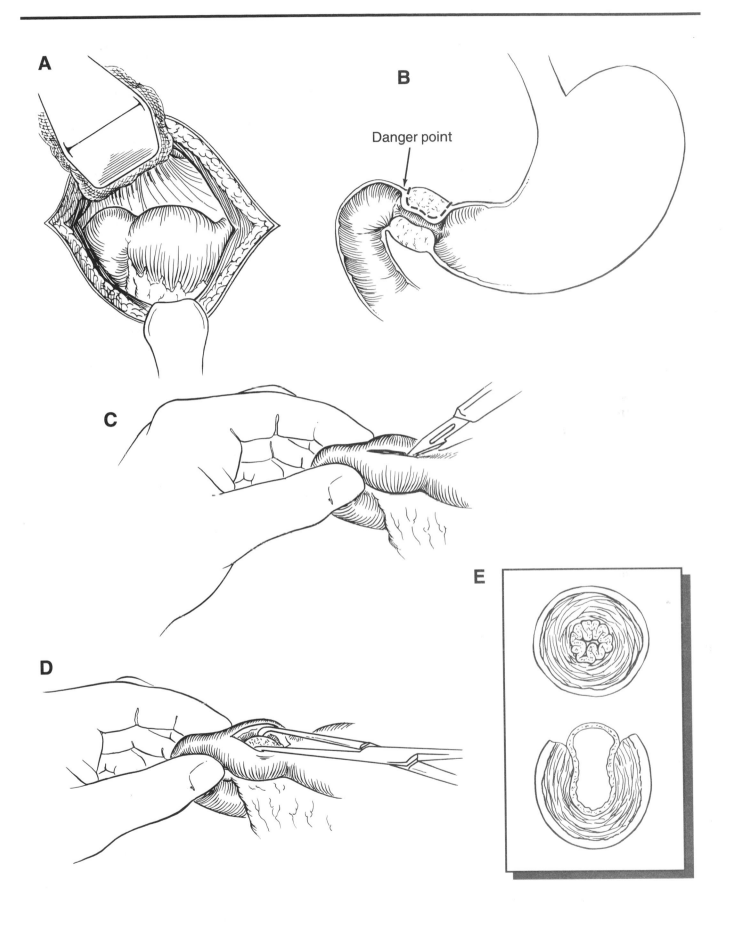

A

B

Danger point

C

D

E

Pyloromyotomy for Congenital Hypertrophic Pyloric Stenosis

Nissen Fundoplication
for Reflux Esophagitis
and Gastric Volvulus

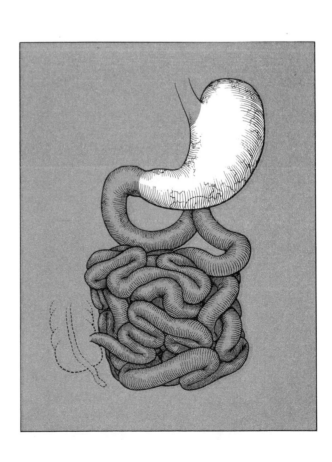

5

Controversy regarding indications for operation in patients who have reflux esophagitis caused by hiatal hernia has been elevated to an art form by zealots and sceptics, medical and surgical. The relative importance of symptomatology, of anatomic changes, of monitored alterations in pressure and pH as primary indicators for therapy—all have their champions. Some gastroenterologists are intensely interested in gastroesophageal reflux disease (GERD) and many claim high degrees of therapeutic success, with only occasional failures who are referred for surgical operation. The great interest in transthoracic repair of hiatal hernia appears to be waning, perhaps because most thoracic surgeons are now preoccupied with the heart. There are, of course, notable exceptions.

The large numbers of procedures advocated for repair of esophageal reflux provides clear evidence of lack of uniform success. Certain individuals have achieved clearly documented success with individualized operative procedures, for example, the arcuate ligament repair of Hill. Most surgeons now appear to prefer Nissen fundoplication for patients with reflux esophagitis of severity sufficient to merit operative intervention. Nissen himself added anterior-wall gastropexy (attachment of the anterior wall of the stomach to the posterior surface of the anterior abdominal wall under some tension), but this part of the operation has been largely abandoned. Nobody knew exactly how much tension to place—if there was too much, the stomach tore away and often leaked, and if there was not enough, the effort was wasted.

All controversy aside, it should probably be noted that the frequency of operation for symptomatic hiatal hernia appears to vary greatly in different regions of the country and is highest in areas where surgeons reside who have great interest and enthusiasm for the operative approach to therapy.

I will describe here the technique we utilize for Nissen fundoplication.

FIG 5–1

A.   The esophagus is mobilized as shown (see Chapter 11). Placement of the Penrose drain around the gastroesophageal junction allows traction that will pull the esophagus down out of the hernia. The large opening in the esophageal hiatus should be narrowed by placement of sutures in the medial and lateral divisions of the right diaphragmatic crus. This illustration shows a large (no. 40 to 48 F) Maloney dilator which has been passed through the patient's mouth into the stomach by the anesthesiologist. The dilator will protect against narrowing of the lumen during fundoplication.

B.   Nearly every study has shown that narrowing the hiatal aperture is, by itself, ineffective in preventing esophageal reflux, but most surgeons continue to perform this part of the procedure, probably because it is easy to do and may help. As shown, we use three heavy (0 polyglactin [Vicryl]) sutures, we have a no. 40 F Maloney dilator in the esophagus, and we leave sufficient space in the hiatus for the tip of the fifth finger.

C.   Traction is maintained on the esophagus by means of a sling of a Penrose drain pulling on the distal esophagus with the inlying no. 40 F Maloney dilator. The intra-abdominal esophagus and proximal stomach are thoroughly freed from all peritoneal attachments and the uppermost three or four sets of vasa brevia connecting the gastric fundus and the superior pole of the spleen are divided and ligated. The proximal stomach should be free of all circumferential attachments, so as to allow free movement proximally, up and around the esophagus, without tension. I often find that insufficient attention is given to this step, especially to posterior mobilization, which leads to difficulty in bringing up enough of the stomach to wrap easily around the esophagus.

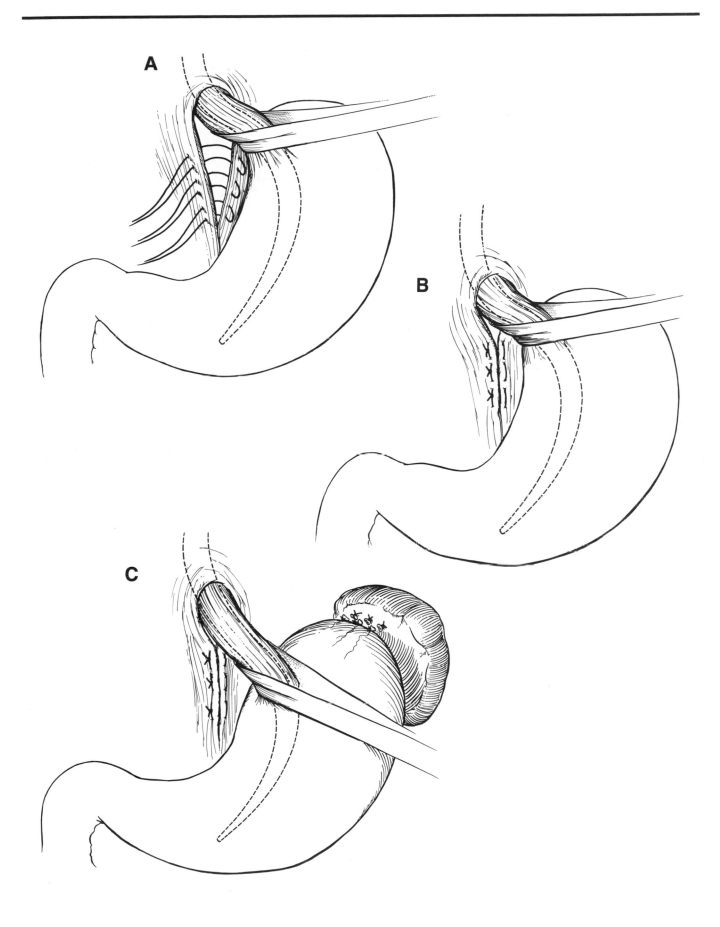

D. The posterior wall of the stomach is coaxed and pulled up behind the esophagus. This is facilitated by straight distal traction on the Penrose drain, which fixes the cardia as the fundus is pulled upwards around the intra-abdominal esophagus. The walls of the stomach are grasped with Allis forceps and held loosely around the esophagus. If approximation is tight, the stomach should be further mobilized. Avoid excess tension on the clamps. Three or four interrupted heavy sutures (0 or 2-0 polyglactin) are placed through the stomach on both sides of the esophagus, so as to hold the wall of the stomach around the esophagus. Most surgeons take a bite of the anterior wall of the esophagus with the suture so as to mitigate against slippage of the esophagus. I am not sure that is effective, but it is well established by tradition. The number of sutures and the length of the wrap vary. We usually place about three or four sutures 1 cm apart, being sure that they are so placed as to allow approximation of the anterior wall of the stomach around the esophagus without tension.

E. The completed Nissen fundoplication reestablishes the esophagogastric junction by bringing the stomach up and wrapping it around the intra-abdominal esophagus, preventing the intra-abdominal esophagus from sliding up into the thorax. Complaints of inability to belch (so-called "gas bloat") after the Nissen procedure can be diminished by leaving the large Maloney dilator in the stomach during the procedure so as to preserve the lumen. Even so, however, many people complain of postoperative distention and inability to belch. A surprising fact to many critical surgeons is that relief of symptoms is not entirely correlated with successful repair. That is, some patients in whom Nissen fundoplication is disrupted anatomically and whose barium radiographs show clear reflux postoperatively will have scant symptoms. Other patients will have return of symptoms with no evidence of reflux. In such instances, we again resort to medical measures in an attempt to manage the situation without reoperation.

F. There is certainly no argument that surgical correction is required for the rare complication of gastric volvulus, in which the stomach herniates into the chest, twisting on either its horizontal or vertical axis.

G. The stomach should be gently reduced by manual traction, delivered into the abdominal cavity, and untwisted. Reduction is usually surprisingly simple. Closing the enlarged hiatus (shown in **A** and **B**) is especially important in these patients; the repair is completed with a Nissen fundoplication.

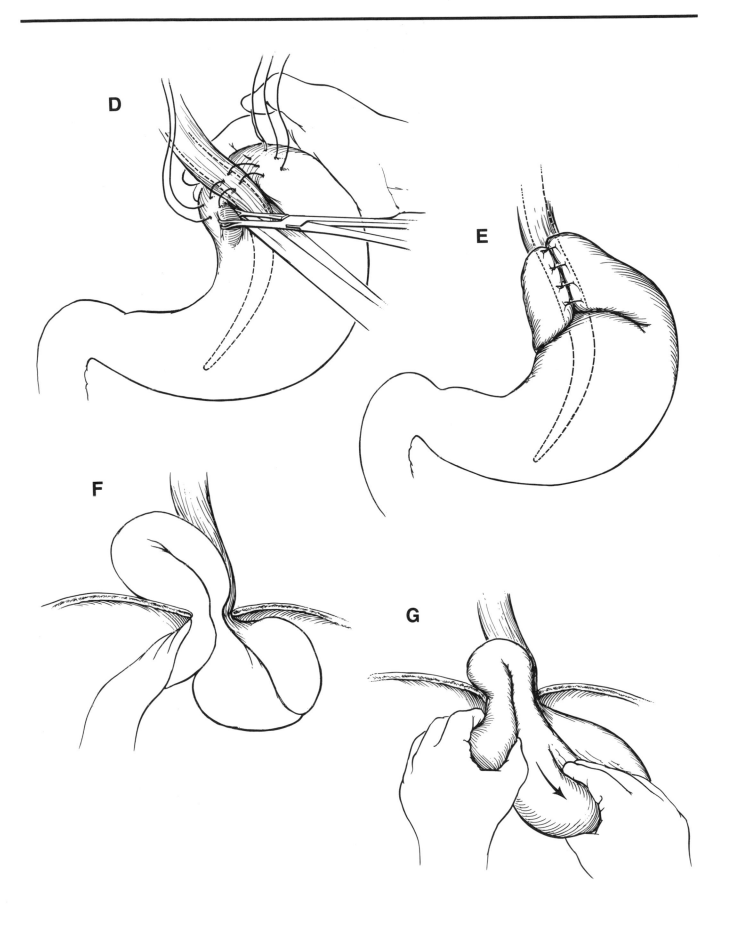

Stomach Trauma

6

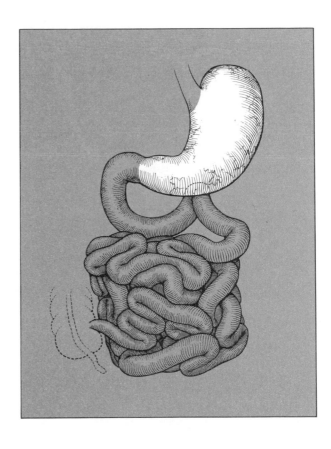

The stomach may be injured by external trauma (either blunt or penetrating) or by trauma from within the lumen caused by endoscopy, by ingestion of caustic substances, by nasogastric tubes, or by sword swallowing. Patients who swallow caustics (such as lye, NaOH [in such proprietary agents as Plumber's Helper], strong ammonia, or battery acid) may require extraordinary care. Ingestion of caustic bases (lye, sodium hydroxide, or strong ammonia solutions) usually causes injury to the pharynx and esophagus; rarely is the stomach greatly injured unless large amounts are ingested. Acid, conversely, may cause relatively minor injuries to the mouth, pharynx, and esophagus, and yet destroy the gastric mucosa and produce full-thickness necrosis of the stomach. Any patient who has swallowed any caustic substance should be followed up with the realization that the patient is at risk for major injury to the esophagus and stomach.

In managing patients with penetrating injuries to the stomach, the extent of injury is usually fairly clear at operation, but the surgeon should be alert to the possibility of a missed injury to the posterior wall of the stomach. Some penetrating injuries appear tangential on the anterior wall and yet may have injured the posterior wall because of approximation.

FIG 6−1

A. The extent of injury to the stomach by gunshot wounds is, of course, a function of the size and muzzle velocity of the missile. High-velocity missiles (from hunting rifles or military weapons) create a large zone of injury around the actual site of penetration and emergence, and tissue must be carefully debrided so as not to leave areas of necrosis. We routinely convert all entrance and exit wounds into small gastrotomies so as to inspect the site of the injury and then close them with a Connell suture, and reinforce this with a layer of interrupted 4-0 polyglactin (Vicryl) sutures. A major problem in most gunshot wounds of the stomach is the high probability of injury to adjacent organs, liver, pancreas, small bowel, spleen, and colon (or heart or lungs). When inspecting the stomach, it is important to divide the gastrohepatic and gastrocolic ligaments so as to allow full inspection of the posterior wall of the stomach. Massive injuries caused by close-proximity shotgun blasts may require massive debridement and extensive resection. If the patient's condition is critical, it may be wise to totally excise the stomach (if indicated), staple the ends of the duodenum and esophagus, and plan to do a Roux-en-Y esophagojejunostomy some days later when the patient's improved condition warrants repair.

B. In many clinics, including our own, patients with knife wounds of the abdomen without signs of peritonitis and with stable vital signs are followed expectantly without immediate operation. Most people with gastric wounds will, of course, manifest physical evidence of peritoneal irritation, but occasionally leaks will occur into the retrogastric space but not manifest clear physical signs for several hours. Large knife wounds of the distal stomach or lesser curvature may prove difficult to close without compromising the lumen. Partial gastrectomy may prove necessary. Necrotic devascularized mucosa should be debrided before closing and the stomach should be emptied. If the knife wound has clearly divided the gastrohepatic ligament, severing the nerves of Latarjet, consideration should be given to truncal vagotomy and gastric drainage (either gastrojejunostomy or pyloroplasty, since the injury may have denervated the antrum, which is the pump that empties the stomach).

C. Blunt injury may result in blowout perforations of the stomach, which may occur anywhere. The injury may be readily accessible or may occur posteriorly or high on the fundus, as shown here.

D. Blowout injuries may occur along the greater curvature. The surgeon should carefully examine the entire bowel. We had a patient who was working under a conveyor belt at a dry dock when the belt broke and dropped, successively, twenty 50-lb sacks of sand onto his chest and abdomen, causing blow-out perforations of his stomach and esophagus.

E. After careful mobilization and after securing hemostasis, the wound is closed with a running Connell inverting suture of 3−0 or 4−0 polyglactin. Here the greater omentum has been dissected away so as to afford clear exposure.

F. The through-and-through running Connell stitch is then reinforced with a row of interrupted 4-0 polyglactin sutures. We usually reinforce the closure with a tab of omentum.

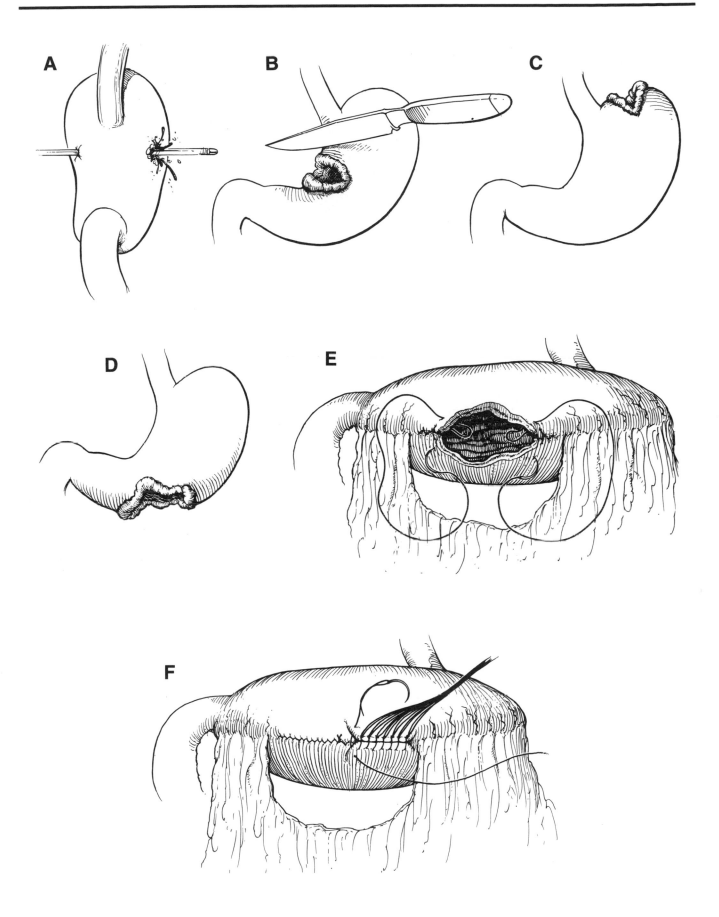

Subtotal Gastrectomy With Billroth I Anastomosis (Also Resection for Benign Distal Gastric Ulcer)

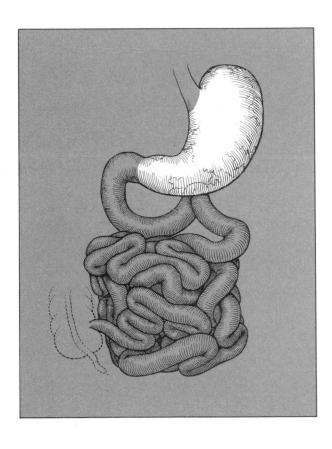

7

Subtotal gastrectomy was first successfully performed by Theodor Billroth at the Allegemeine Krankenhaus in Vienna in 1881. The procedure was first performed in a patient who had a malignant obstruction of the pylorus. After performing what was actually an extended pylorectomy, Billroth reestablished gut continuity by anastomosing the stomach to the duodenum. Von Rydigier adapted subtotal gastrectomy with gastroduodenostomy for treatment of duodenal ulcer disease in 1882. Later, after subtotal gastric resection in another patient, Billroth reestablished continuity by means of a gastrojejunostomy, after closing the duodenal stump just distal to the pylorus.

FIG 7–1

A. Subtotal gastrectomy now is used to treat patients with duodenal ulcer disease, gastric ulcer disease, gastric cancer, trauma, gastritis, and benign neoplasms. A principle of the procedure is that all of the antral mucosa is taken so that the duodenum is divided beyond the pylorus, shown here as the distal dotted line. The proximal line of division varies according to the extent of resection required. (Resection at the top dotted line, for example, provides a 75% distal gastrectomy.) After removal of the distal stomach, continuity can be restored either by gastroduodenostomy (Billroth I) or gastrojejunostomy (Billroth II). In patients operated on for peptic ulcer disease, the procedure can be used alone or in conjunction with vagotomy. Resection combined with vagotomy is used chiefly in treatment of complications of duodenal ulcer. When combined with vagotomy, resection is limited to 40% to 50% of the distal stomach. Operations for gastric ulcer usually do not include vagotomy. When the operation is performed for gastric cancer, any required amount of the stomach may be resected (60% to 80%, up to a total gastrectomy).

B. In the event that the subtotal gastrectomy is to be performed on a patient with a gastric ulcer or with a purportedly benign neoplasm, and if the patient has not already undergone endoscopic biopsy to determine whether the ulcer or the tumor is malignant, the patient should have an intraoperative biopsy with frozen section. This illustration shows initiation of the gastrotomy. If the ulcer or neoplasm is on the anterior wall of the stomach, the gastrotomy should of course be placed away from the lesion.

C. After establishing the line of the gastrotomy by partial-thickness electrocautery incision, the lumen is entered with a right-angle clamp and the remaining thickness of the gastric wall tented with the blades of the instrument open, so as to afford access by electrocautery to complete the gastrotomy without mucosal bleeding. This technique for gastrotomy is often useful in patients who have great pyloric deformity because of ulcer disease. It is frequently helpful to determine the direction of the pyloric channel, to palpate the duodenal ulcer, and to ascertain the position of the ampulla of Vater, which is often pulled in a proximal direction by scarring. Palpation of the ampulla may require a more distal extension of the gastrotomy wound.

D. This illustrates biopsy of a gastric ulcer located on the posterior wall of the stomach. Most benign gastric ulcers are located on the lesser curvature itself at the incisura angularis.

E. This shows the proper performance of a biopsy for a gastric ulcer. A biopsy taken of the base of the ulcer itself will usually yield only necrotic debris; the tissue removed should contain some normal gastric mucosa, the overhanging edge of the ulcer, and the edge of the ulcer crater.

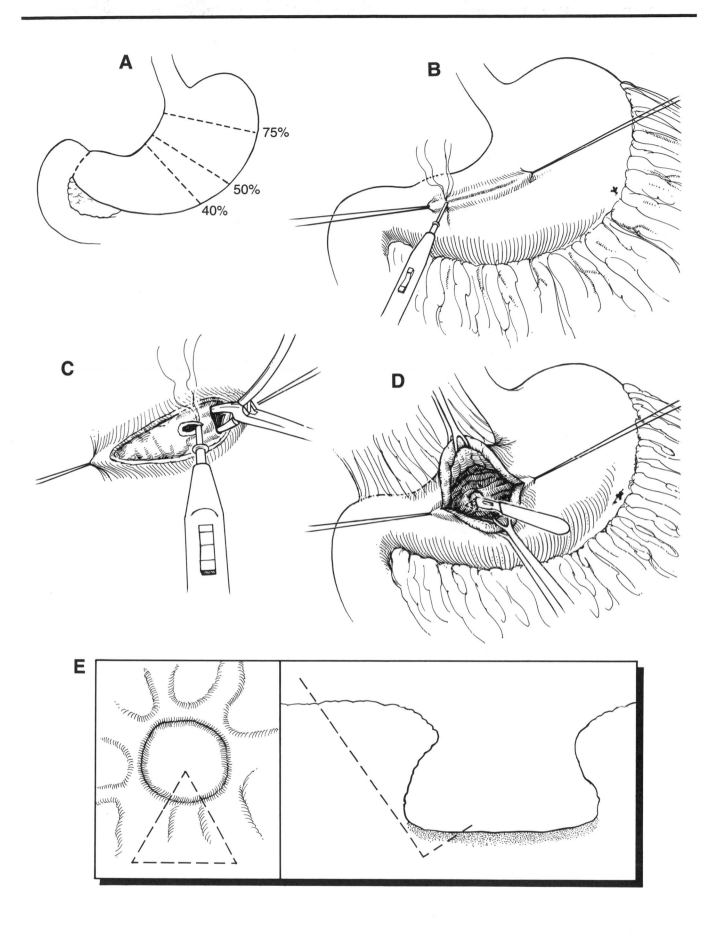

F. The next step in the subtotal gastrectomy is mobilization of the greater curvature of the stomach by serial division of the gastric branches of the gastroepiploic vessels. (This shows closure of the anterior gastrotomy used to biopsy the gastric ulcer. If the resection were for duodenal ulcer disease, there would be no gastrotomy, unless one had been made to facilitate palpation of the pylorus.) The lesser curvature is immobilized by serially dividing the gastrohepatic ligament along the dotted line. Care should be exercised in mobilizing the greater curvature so as to avoid injury to the middle colic vessels. Inflammation will often bind the gastrocolic ligament to the transverse mesocolon, and it may be necessary to carefully dissect the middle colic vessels away from the gastrocolic ligament.

G. The left gastric vessels are identified, clamped, and ligated.

H. After the lesser curvature has been mobilized proximal to the left gastric artery and distal to the gastroduodenal artery, two large Payr clamps are placed across the line of proximal division of the stomach. A small Payr clamp (barely shown) is then placed across the greater curvature just proximal to the proximal large Payr clamp. The tissue within the small Payr will serve as the gastric orifice for the anastomosis. The distal line of division should be beyond the pylorus, which is usually clearly marked by the palpable ring of muscle and by the veins of Mayo. Mobilization of the proximal duodenum in patients with duodenal ulcer disease or with pyloric channel peptic ulcer may be difficult. A Kocher maneuver is helpful. The distal stomach should be swung anteriorly to the right, and distal traction placed so as to facilitate dissection of the posterior wall of the distal stomach and proximal duodenum away from the head of the pancreas.

I. After the distal stomach is fully mobilized, the proximal duodenum is divided between large Kocher clamps on a line just distal to the pylorus, shown here by the dotted line.

J. The closure of the lesser curvature side of the proximal line of division of the stomach is of crucial importance, since leaks have disastrous consequences. The method shown here takes a bit of time, but has proven to be safe and effective. A 0 polyglactin (Vicryl) suture on a swaged needle is placed back and forth behind the large Payr clamp in a basting stitch. This suture line is carried to the tip of the small Payr clamp; the large Payr is then removed.

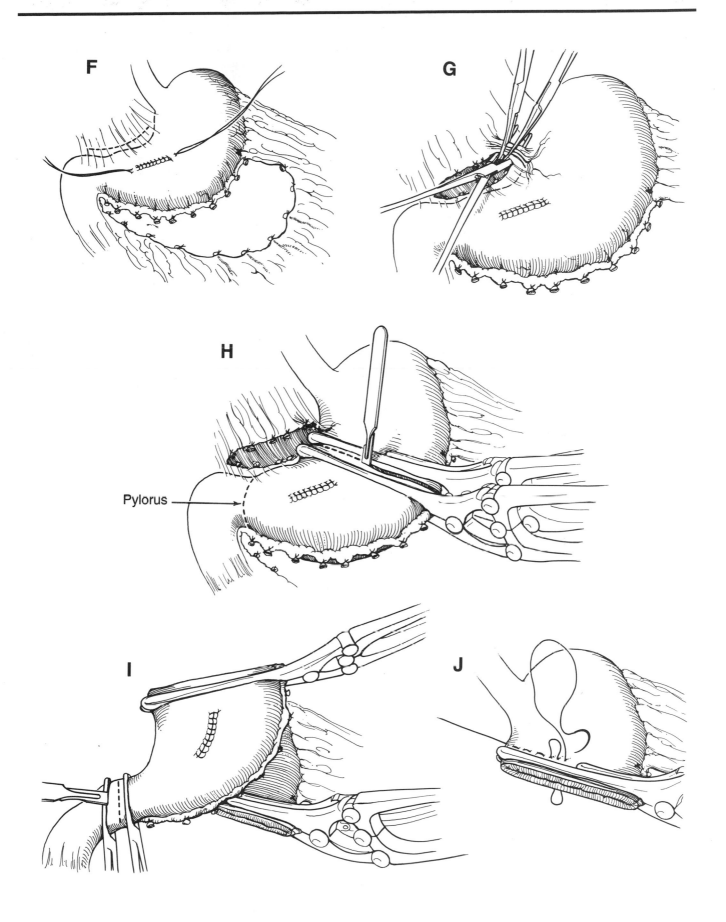

F

G

H

Pylorus

I

J

Subtotal Gastrectomy With Billroth I Anastomosis

K. The crushed tissue is excised from in front of the jaws of the small Payr clamp and anterior to the basted suture line. The suture is then tied just anterior to the jaw of the small Payr clamp.

L. The suture line is then carried toward the lesser curvature in a running locking fashion to achieve hemostasis.

M. The suture line is then inverted with a running Lembert suture after first inverting the lesser curvature corner of the suture line with a hemipursestring suture. Gastrointestinal continuity can then be restored by anastomosing the stomach either to the duodenum or jejunum.

N. In a Billroth I anastomosis, the clamp holding the cut end of the duodenum is approximated to the small Payr clamp on the greater curvature of the stomach and a posterior row of interrupted 4-0 polyglactin sutures is placed so as to approximate the posterior walls of the stomach and duodenum. After tying, all sutures are cut except the two ends, which will be used as stay sutures for the rest of the anastomosis.

O. After removal of the clamps from the stomach and duodenum, the crushed redundant mucosa is excised with the cautery and all bleeding points are clamped with mosquito clamps and tied with 4-0 sutures. It is important to achieve complete hemostasis in this manner and not to depend on the continuous suture.

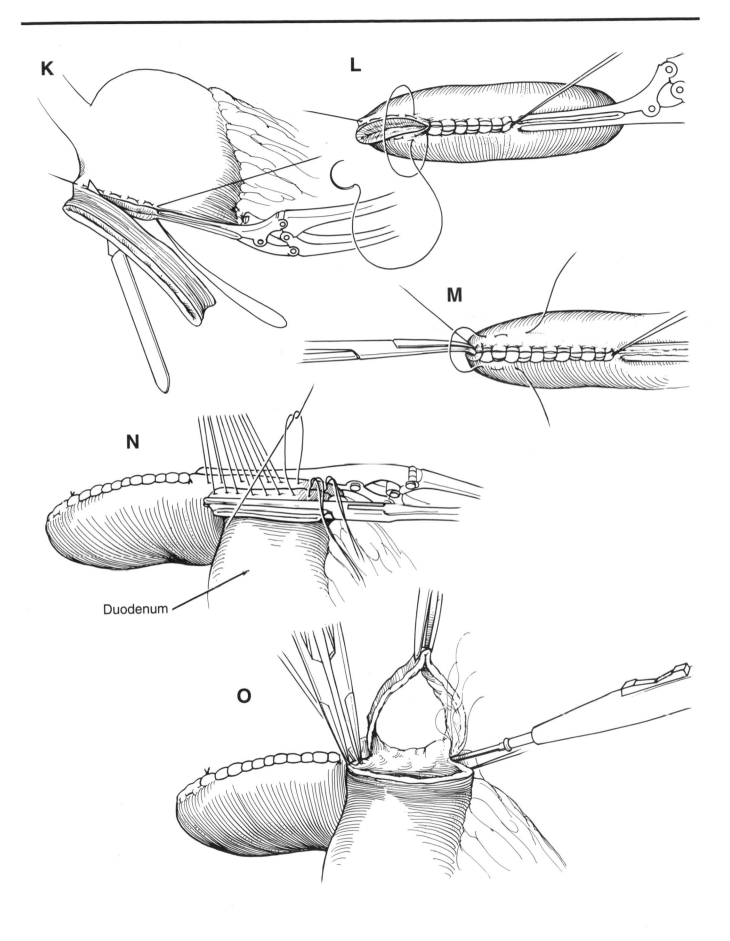

K

L

M

N

Duodenum

O

P. After removal of the small Payr clamp, the lumen of the gastric side of the anastomosis is almost always larger than the duodenal side. This discrepancy can be corrected, if necessary, by excising a V-shaped wedge from the anterior wall of the duodenum.

Q. The anastomosis is continued by placement of two swaged 4-0 polyglactin sutures adjacent to one another on the posterior row, tying the short ends together and cutting them. Each suture is then carried away from the other in a running locking posterior row. At the end of the posterior row, the sutures are brought out and the corner is turned by converting to a running Connell suture, which provides a continuous inverting row.

R. The continuous Connell suture is carried around anteriorly and the two sutures are tied together. The anterior suture line is then reinforced with an interrupted serosal row of 4-0 polyglactin sutures.

S. The suture line may be covered by a tab of omentum brought up and tied in place anteriorly. We rarely do this. This figure shows a completed 50% distal gastrectomy and gastroduodenostomy.

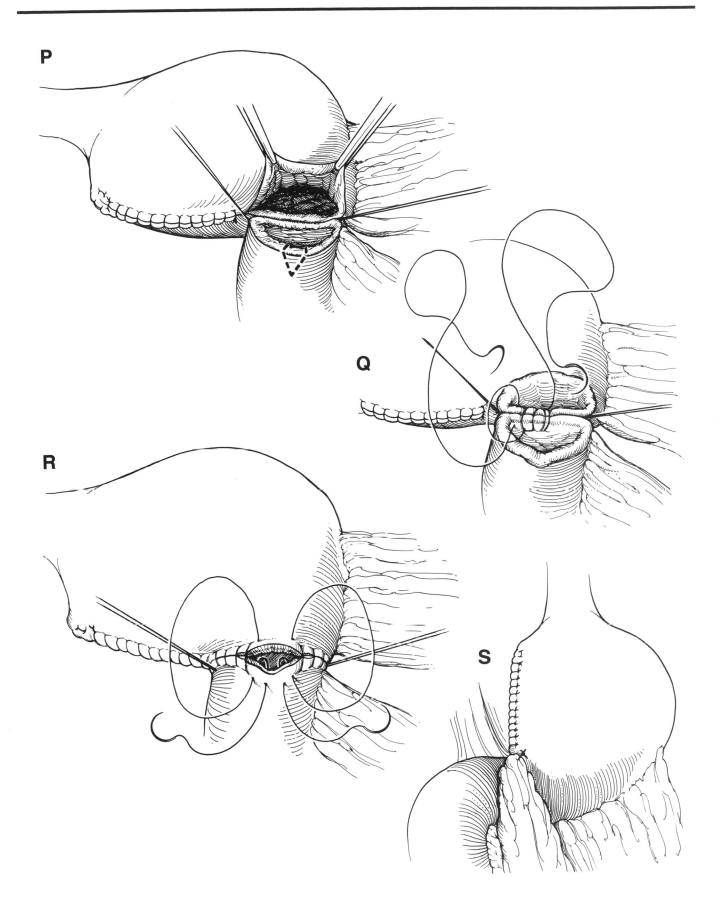

P

Q

R

S

Subtotal Gastrectomy With Stapled Billroth I Anastomosis

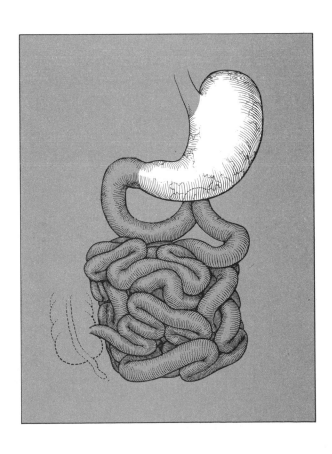

8

An alternative to the hand-sewn gastroduodenostomy (shown in Chapter 7) is the performance of a stapled anastomosis between the stomach and duodenum. Practical application is relatively limited, since the duodenum must be sufficiently pliable so as to be anastomosed safely by means of the end-to-end stapling device. Such a situation, of course, is present in patients with benign gastric ulcer who have undergone distal subtotal gastrectomy.

FIG 8–1

A. The distal portion of the stomach is mobilized (see Chapter 7) and the duodenum divided between Kocher clamps just distal to the pylorus. A site for division of the stomach is selected and a large double-row stapling device is placed and fired, and the stomach divided between the proximal stapling device and large Kocher clamps placed across the greater and lesser curvature, as shown. The duodenum is divided just distal to the pylorus between Kocher clamps.

B. This shows the divided stapled proximal stomach. Stay sutures are inserted and traction exerted on the anterior gastric wall just proximal to the staple line. An aperture is made with the electrocautery through the anterior wall of the stomach.

C. The GIA stapling device is then inserted through the aperture into the stomach and fired, so as to divide the anterior gastric wall between two rows of staples.

D. The EEA stapling device with the post extended is then inserted into the stomach through the stapled gastrotomy. The post is then pressed against the posterior wall, the serosa of the posterior wall is scored with the electrocautery, and the post is pushed through.

A

B

C

D

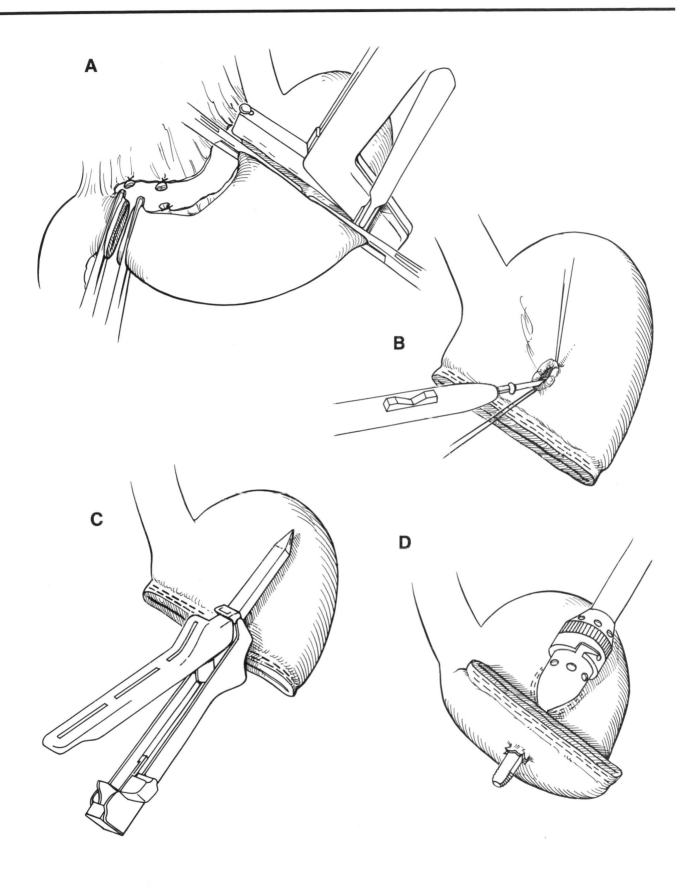

E. The clamp is removed from the duodenum and three stay sutures applied. After hemostasis is secured in the wall of the duodenum, a pursestring suture of heavy prolene is placed circumferentially around the proximal duodenum. The anvil is then attached to the post of the EEA and inserted into the duodenal lumen. The pursestring suture is then tightened and tied, so as to secure the anvil within the duodenum.

F. The anvil and the EEA stapling device are approximated by turning the thumbscrew at the base of the stapler. The EEA device is then fired, the anvil and head are separated and distracted by extending the post using the thumbscrew, and the anvil is gently retracted through the gastroduodenostomy anastomosis and out the stapled gastrotomy wound.

G. This figure shows the stapled anastomosis between the duodenum and posterior gastric wall. The stapled gastrotomy wound is closed by grasping the edges of the wound with Babcock forceps; the TA-55 stapling device is placed so as to close the wound. The device is approximated and fired and the excess tissue excised.

H. This figure shows the completed anastomosis with the stapled gastroduodenostomy between the proximal duodenum and the posterior wall of the stomach, the stapled distal end of the divided stomach, and the stapled aperture through which the EEA stapling device was placed.

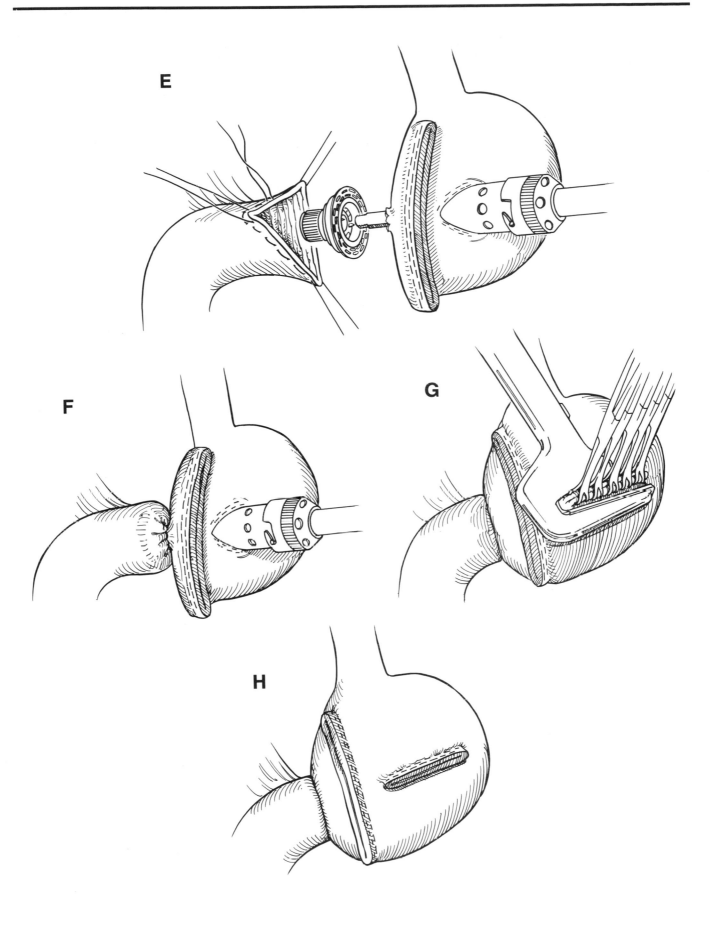

E

F

G

H

Subtotal Gastrectomy With Billroth II Anastomosis

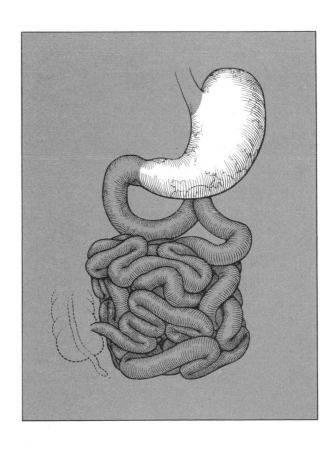

9

The choice between gastroduodenostomy (Billroth I) and gastrojejunostomy (Billroth II) in restoring continuity of the gut after subtotal gastric resection is largely idiosyncratic; that is, it usually depends upon the experience of the surgeon. There does seem to be good evidence, mainly from experience at the Mayo Clinic, that the Billroth II subtotal gastrectomy for duodenal ulcer disease has a lower rate of ulcer recurrence than does the Billroth I, provided that the vagus is intact. In patients who have had antrectomy plus truncal vagotomy for duodenal ulcer, however, most studies have shown the Billroth I hook-up to be superior. The usual explanation is that duodenal mechanisms for inhibition of acid secretion remain in continuity with the Billroth I procedure.

On the other hand, in operations for cancer of the distal stomach, most surgeons prefer the Billroth II anastomosis, since local recurrence of the cancer would tend to cause earlier obstruction of a gastroduodenostomy. In performing the Billroth II anastomosis, the choice of whether the jejunal loop is brought anterior to the transverse colon or brought posteriorly through the transverse mesocolon is largely a matter of personal preference.

FIG 9–1

A. This illustration shows an approximate 50% distal subtotal gastric resection with the Payr clamps in place and after a stapled closure of the proximal duodenum just distal to the pylorus. If the duodenum is badly scarred, many surgeons would avoid a stapled closure, because of the thick, scarred, ischemic duodenal wall. In such an instance, hand-sewn closure of the duodenum (**G–J**) is probably to be preferred. Shown here, the duodenum is divided between the pylorus and the stapled suture line and the distal stomach delivered from the wound. In this procedure, a segment of jejunum approximately 12 to 15 cm distal to the ligament of Treitz is selected and brought anterior to the transverse colon for a gastrojejunal anastomosis.

B. This figure shows the posterior row of interrupted polyglactin sutures tied in place between the stomach and jejunum. The gastric stoma is held by the Payr clamps and the jejunal stoma will be made by electrocautery dissection along the dotted line.

C. This figure shows the closure of the anterior wall of the anastomosis by means of Connell sutures using two 4-0 swaged polyglactin (Vicryl) sutures.

D. This figure shows the completed 50% subtotal gastric resection with antecolic gastrojejunostomy and stapled duodenal stump.

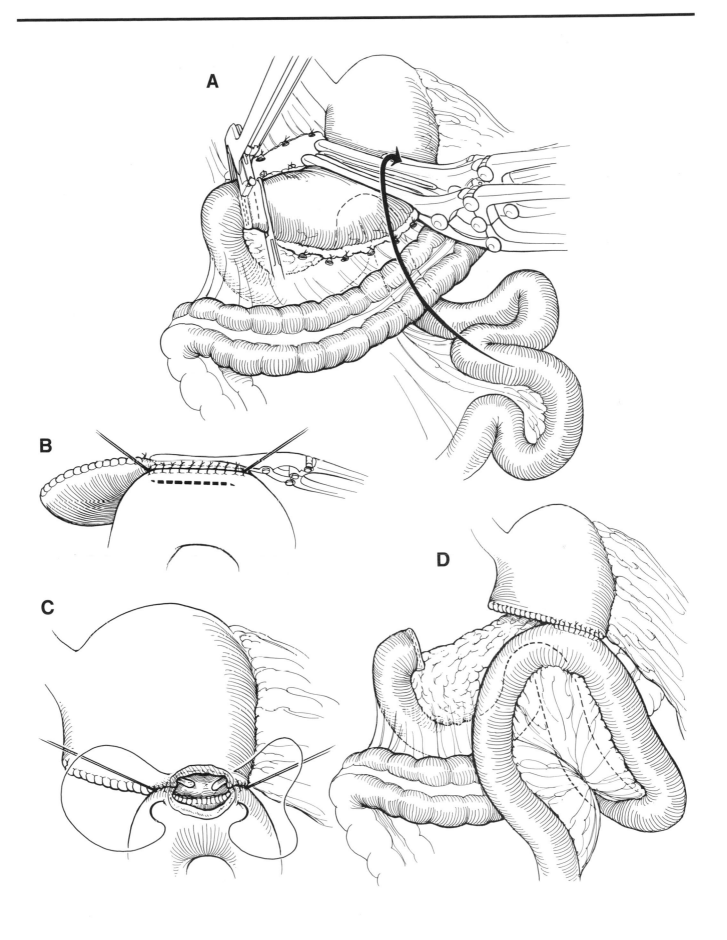

E. This figure shows the alternative method of posterior gastrojejunostomy, in which an opening is made in the transverse mesocolon (taking care to avoid vessels from the middle colic artery going to the colon). A routine two-layer anastomosis is created between the stomach and the jejunum.

F. This figure shows completion of the anastomosis with closure of the rent in the transverse mesocolon so as to prevent herniation of the small bowel.

G. As previously mentioned, if the duodenum is badly scarred, the stapled closure may not be safe. In this instance, an alternative is to suture the duodenal stump. In this instance, the duodenum has been divided and the end held in place with a Kocher clamp. The initial closure is performed with a basting stitch of 4-0 polyglactin swaged suture, behind the jaws of the Kocher clamp.

H. The clamp has been removed and the redundant tissue excised.

I. Each end of the suture line is then inverted with a hemipursestring suture.

J. The closure is then completed with an interrupted row of polyglactin sutures.

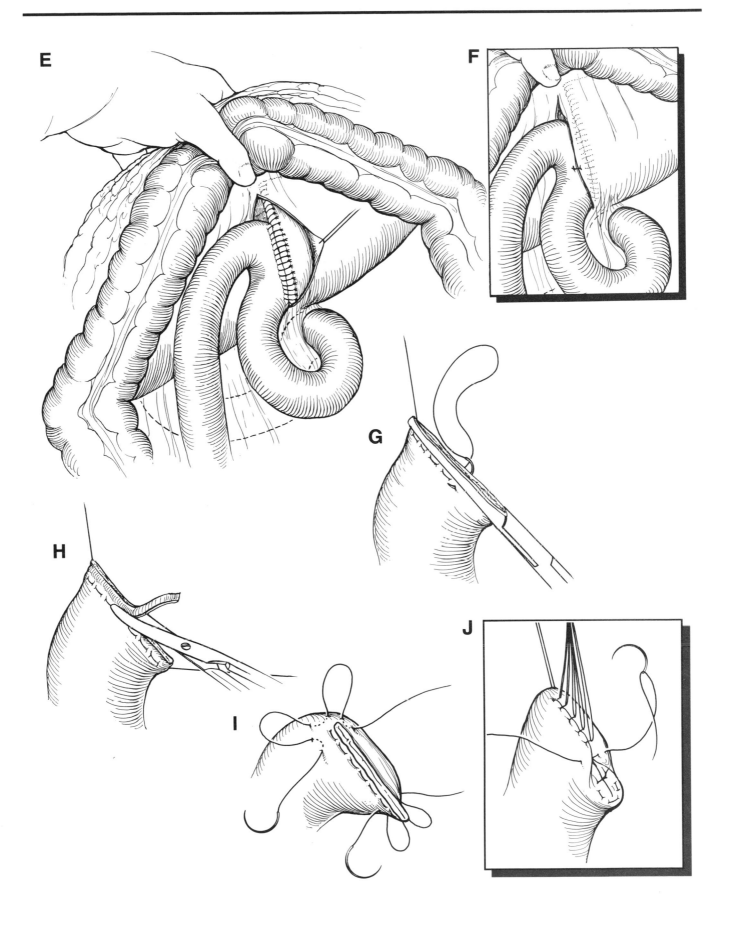

Subtotal Gastrectomy With Stapled Billroth II Anastomosis

10

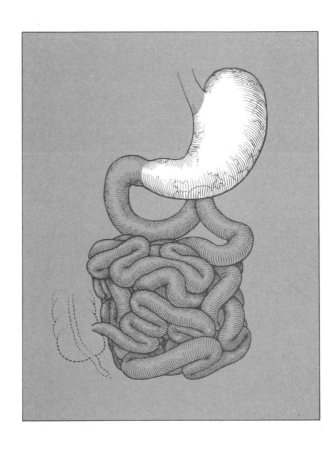

An alternative method for performance of the gastrojejunostomy in the Billroth II distal subtotal gastrectomy is to perform the anastomoses with stapling devices. The choice between a stapled and a hand-sewn anastomosis is clearly influenced by personal experience. I often use staples on the esophagus, small bowel, and colon, but I prefer not to use them on the stomach because of the great thickness of the gastric wall. I know, however, that many successful surgeons routinely perform stapled gastrojejunostomies.

FIG 10–1

A.   In this instance, the distal stomach has been dissected and the pylorus divided between a staple line just distal to the pylorus and a clamp (see Fig **9–1, A,** p. 63). This figure shows the distal stomach dissected free and elevated anteriorly by means of a Payr clamp placed across the distal stomach at the pylorus. The line of division was just distal to the pylorus. A proximal limb of jejunum has been selected and brought anterior to the transverse mesocolon and brought up so as to approximate the posterior wall of the stomach at a level just proximal to the preselected site of division of the stomach. Apertures have been made into the adjacent walls of the stomach and jejunum with the electrocautery and the two limbs of the GIA stapling device have been inserted so as to approximate the stomach and jejunum. The stapling device is closed and fired and removed, creating a stapled opening between the stomach and jejunum. We place a suture through the serosa of stomach and jejunum just distal to the tip of the GIA staple so as to prevent tension on the end of the stapled anastomosis.

B.   The stomach is elevated and a TA-95 stapling device is placed across the distal stomach and also across the jejunal aperture through which the GIA stapling device was inserted. The TA-95 stapler is then fired and the excess stomach and the small jejunal segment are excised.

C.   This illustrates the completed subtotal gastrectomy with stapled antecolic gastrojejunostomy. The jejunum, of course, can also be brought posterior to the colon through an opening made in the transverse mesocolon so as to create a stapled posterior gastrojejunostomy.

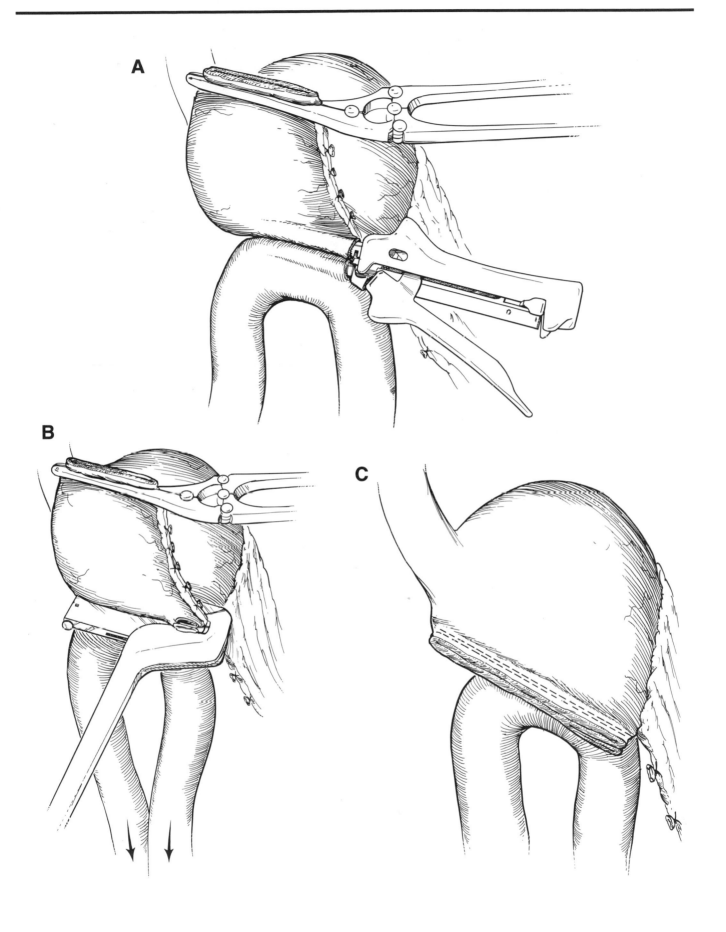

Truncal Vagotomy

11

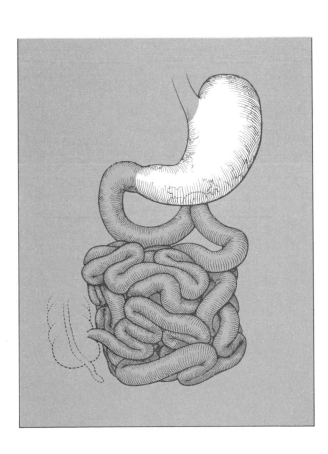

Truncal vagotomy provides a safe and simple means for reducing acid secretion by the stomach. Since the vagus contains two kinds of efferent fibers, one for secretion and one for motility, truncal vagotomy not only inhibits secretion but also diminishes gastric motility, since the vagus provides motor fibers to the circular muscle of the antrum, which is the pump that empties the stomach. Truncal vagotomy must, therefore, be accompanied by a procedure to facilitate gastric drainage; drainage can be achieved by either pyloroplasty or by gastroenterostomy.

The advantages of truncal vagotomy are that it is safe (mortality is low) and many of the serious late postgastrectomy sequelae (severe dumping, bilious vomiting, and nutritional problems) are avoided. The drawbacks to truncal vagotomy lie in the relatively high rate of ulcer recurrence (5% to 8% at 5 years, up to 12% to 15% at 10 to 15 years) and the relatively frequent postoperative sequelae of dumping and diarrhea, both usually mild. Postvagotomy diarrhea is an enigma; vagotomy should achieve an anticholinergic effect, similar to that, say, of atropine, yet atropine paralyzes the bowel. Most postvagotomy diarrhea is mercifully transient and many previously constipated patients look upon it as an unexpected welcome dividend, but about 1% of patients who have undergone truncal vagotomy are sorely troubled for years with diarrhea. The method for vagotomy illustrated here has evolved over 20 years. Careful application will allow simple, safe, reliable vagotomy to be performed in 10 to 12 minutes (more quickly if time is short). We have been very pleased with the results.

FIG 11–1

A. We secure exposure by means of a midline vertical epigastric incision from the xiphoid to just below the umbilicus. A Goligher sternal hook retractor is used to elevate the xiphoid and the wound edges are kept open with a Finochietto-type rib-spreader retractor. The chance of splenic injury can be minimized by putting a sloppy-wet laparotomy pack in the left upper quadrant. Retraction of the left lobe of the liver is achieved with the Weinberg retractor (shown in upper midline), which provides excellent exposure of the esophageal hiatus without dividing the triangular hepatic ligament. The Weinberg retractor ("Joe's hoe") should remain in the midline since lateral drift may injure the spleen.

B. The esophagus is grasped with the right hand lifting it anteriorly. The inlying nasogastric tube facilitates grasping the esophagus.

C. The phrenoesophageal ligament posterior to the esophagus is then broken through either by blunt dissection with fingers or by use of an instrument. Care should be taken to keep all instruments away from contact with the esophagus itself in order to avoid perforation.

D. A medium Penrose drain is then passed around the esophagus for traction. The ends of the drain are clamped with a Mayo clamp, which is then fixed beneath the Finochietto ratchet (not shown). The Penrose places tension on the esophagus and makes the vagal fibers (which are less elastic than the esophagus) more easily palpable.

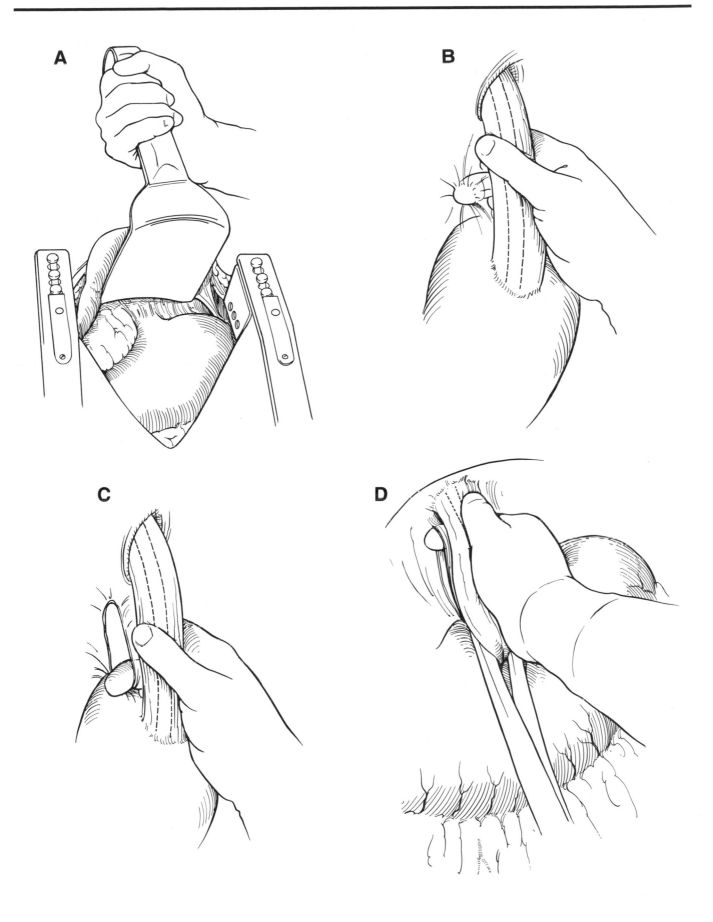

E. By blunt dissection with thumb and forefinger, the reflection of peritoneum onto the esophagus, the phrenoesophageal ligament, is lifted from the surface of the esophagus and the vagal trunks are identified. The anterior trunk is usually located between the 12 o'clock and 2 o'clock positions (xiphoid at 12 o'clock), and the posterior trunk is usually about 6 o'clock to 8 o'clock. The posterior trunk is almost always larger, sometimes three times larger than the anterior. Within the chest, the vagal fibers decussate around the esophagus and often vagal fibers will enter the esophageal musculature above the diaphragm. As a result, complete division of vagus is often impossible (except by esophageal transection). It is important to carry the dissection in a proximal direction to the esophageal hiatus of the diaphragm so that all of the intra-abdominal esophagus is exposed. In performing selective vagotomy procedures, the vagal trunks are identified, tagged with long heavy sutures, and left in place.

F. In performing a truncal vagotomy, we place small metal clips on the vagus and excise a 2-cm segment between the clips. Excised vagal segments are sent for pathologic examination of permanent sections (not for frozen section).

G. The procedure is repeated for the larger posterior nerve. Care should be taken to identify and divide any accessory vagal fibers. As many as five accessory vagal trunks have been reported, but the great majority of individuals have only two main trunks. Traction on the esophagus will often facilitate location of the accessory bundles, since the nerves are less elastic than the muscle fibers. Digging into the muscular wall of the esophagus with a clamp should be avoided, since perforation may result. We usually perform vagotomy prior to resection or performance of a drainage operation (gastrojejunostomy or pyloroplasty). When the entire procedure is complete, the area of the esophageal hiatus should be carefully reinspected for bleeding. We usually manage bleeding vessels of the esophageal wall with small metal clips.

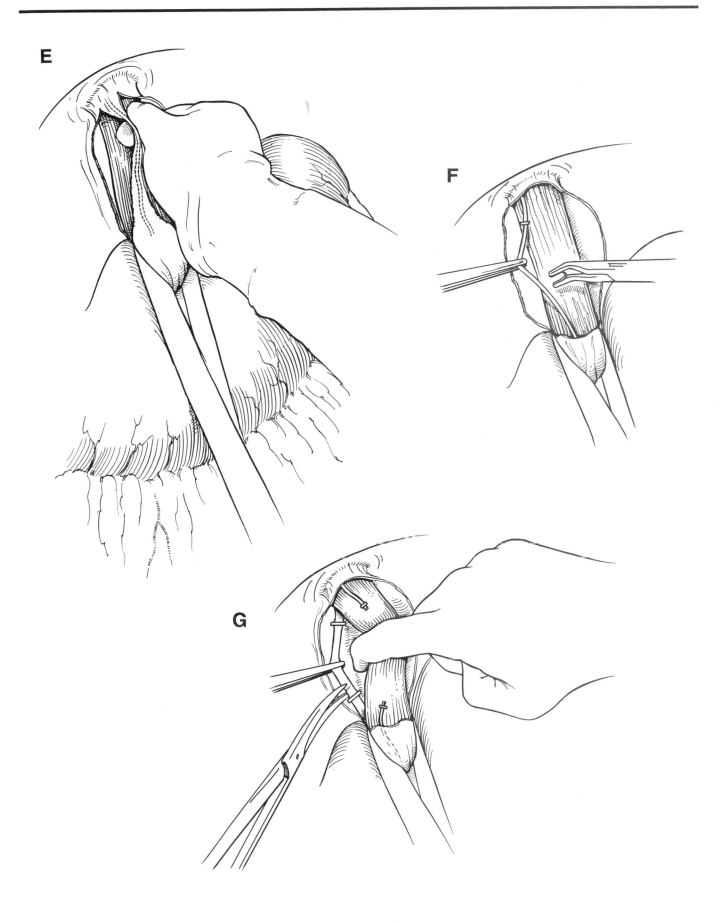

E

F

G

Gastrojejunostomy

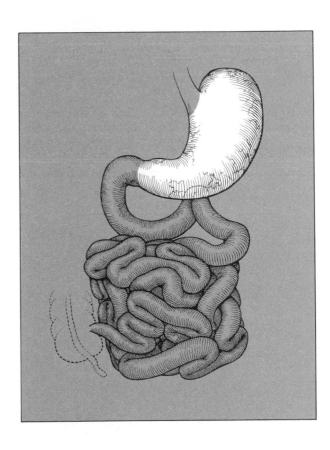

12

Anastomosis between the stomach and proximal jejunum is used to facilitate gastric emptying or to reestablish continuity of the gut after partial gastrectomy. Historically, it was the first surgical procedure used for the empiric treatment of peptic ulcer disease, but ultimately failed because it does not suppress gastric secretion. We usually use gastrojejunostomy now to facilitate gastric drainage in patients who have undergone truncal vagotomy. I prefer an antecolic anastomosis; that is, the loop of jejunum is brought up in front of the colon. Some surgeons prefer a retrocolic gastrojejunostomy, in which the loop of jejunum is brought behind the transverse colon through a rent in the transverse mesocolon. No differences in results of the two procedures have been reported. If the retrocolic approach is used, most surgeons loosely suture the edges of the rent in the mesocolon to the jejunum to minimize risk of herniation of a bowel loop.

We believe that it is probably unsafe to do a gastric drainage procedure without vagotomy, although drainage alone is occasionally performed in patients with benign gastric outlet obstruction; the risk of peptic ulceration is high. Conversely, truncal vagotomy should probably always be accompanied by some form of drainage operation. Gastric drainage is often omitted in patients who have vagotomy during esophageal resection for cancer, but there is always a chance that the stomach will fail progressively to empty, and require later drainage.

FIG 12–1

A. In selecting the segment of bowel to be anastomosed to the stomach, care should be taken so as not to inadvertently grasp a distal limb of small bowel. This can easily be avoided by selecting a point (shown at tip of forceps) 15 to 20 cm distal to the ligament of Treitz. The anastomosis can be made either by bringing the jejunum anterior to the transverse colon, or by bringing up a short loop of jejunum through an opening made in the transverse mesocolon. In either event, the distance between the ligament of Treitz and the anastomosis should not be excessively long, nor should the anastomosis be under any tension. A rare but tragic error is to misidentify the loop of bowel and thereby make an anastomosis between the stomach and ileum. Care should be taken to place the gastric stoma as close to the pylorus as possible so as to ensure drainage of the entire stomach.

B. A posterior row of interrupted 4-0 polyglactin (Vicryl) sutures is placed between the gastric and jejunal serosae and the sites of the gastric and jejunal stomas are scored with the electrocautery.

C. The jejunal stoma is created by dissecting through the serosa and muscularis with the electrocautery current, achieving hemostasis as the dissection progresses. Here the mucosa pouts through. An opening is then made in the mucosa and a right-angled clamp is inserted into the lumen.

D. The clamp is opened and elevated.

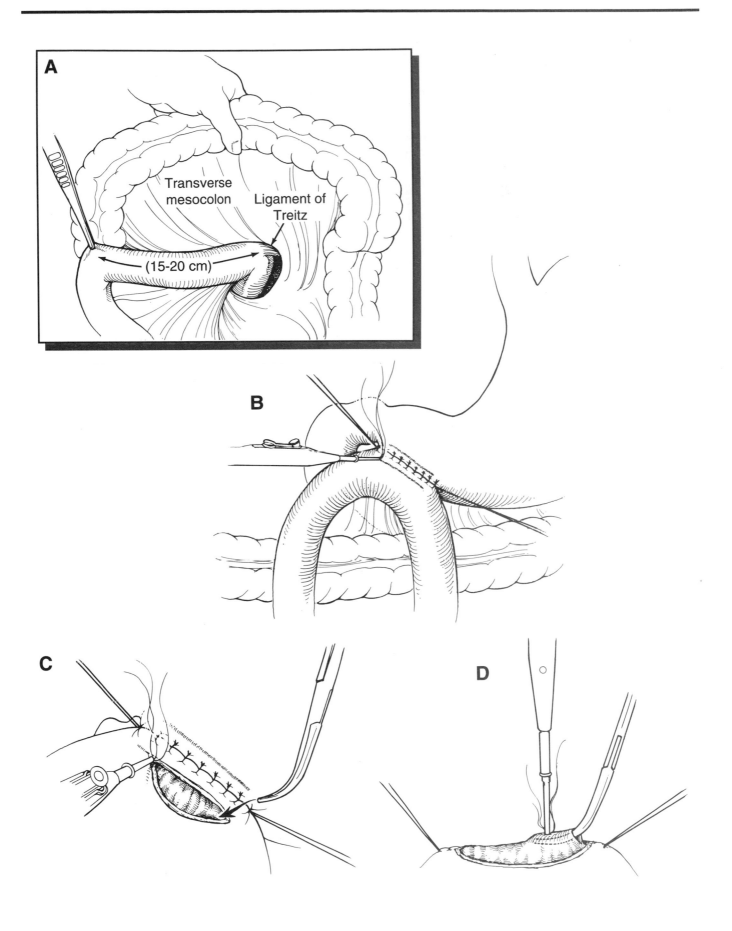

Inside the figures:

A

Transverse mesocolon

Ligament of Treitz

(15-20 cm)

B

C

D

E. The mucosa between the jaws is divided by electrocautery.

F. The procedure is repeated in creating the gastric stoma. This method allows creation of anastomotic stomas without loss of blood and with good protection against postoperative mucosal bleeding.

G. The full-thickness anastomosis is then begun by placing two 4-0 swaged polyglactin sutures posteriorly (in a running locking fashion), and then bringing them around anteriorly as a Connell suture.

H. This shows the completed procedure of truncal vagotomy and antecolic gastrojejunostomy, which allows good drainage of the vagotomized stomach.

I. This shows, for comparison, a completed truncal vagotomy and retrocolic gastrojejunostomy. The retrocolic anastomosis allows for a shorter proximal limb. The opening in the transverse mesocolon should be sewn closed around the jejunal loop.

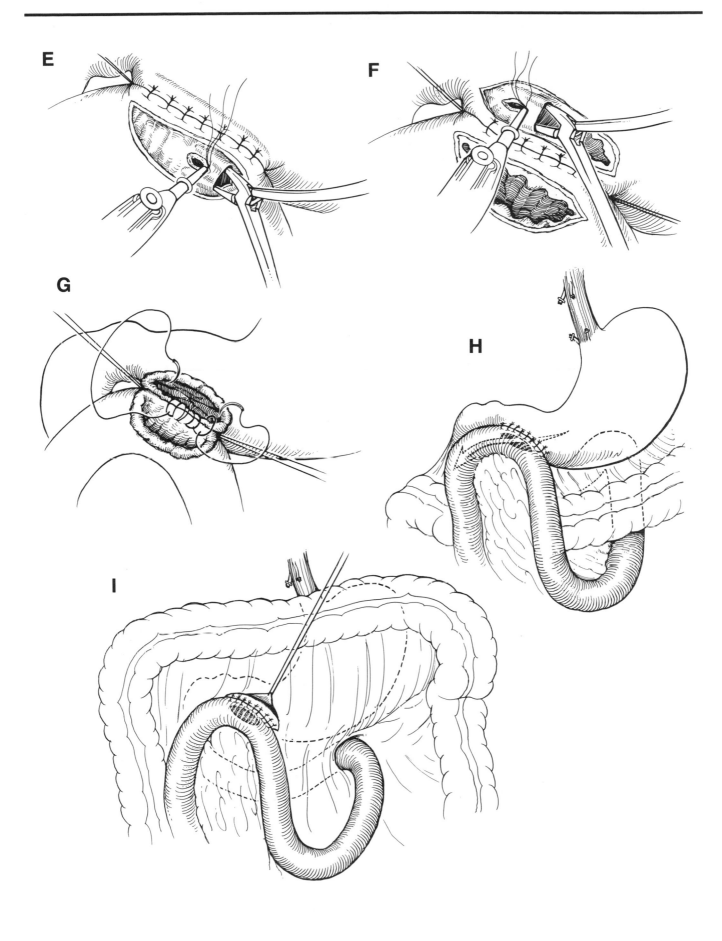

Pyloroplasty

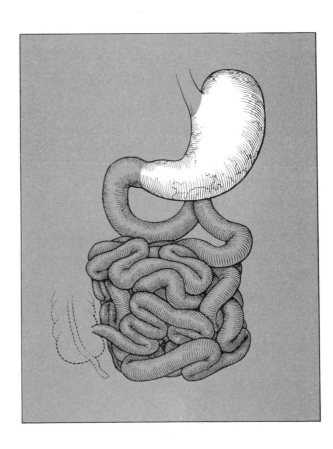

13

Truncal vagotomy denervates the circular smooth muscle of the antrum that acts as the pump that empties the stomach. Truncal vagotomy must, therefore, be complemented by a drainage procedure (which can be provided by either gastrojejunostomy or pyloroplasty). Dragstedt first used gastroenterostomy, and years later, Weinberg adapted the Heineke-Mikulicz pyloroplasty, which enlarges the gastric outlet and facilitates emptying of the denervated stomach. Weinberg's emphasis was on a single-layer closure so as to ensure the largest possible pyloric lumen to facilitate drainage of the denervated stomach.

FIG 13–1

A. The principle, of course, of the Heineke-Mikulicz pyloroplasty is to enlarge the pyloric stoma by means of a transverse incision that is closed vertically. The first step is to perform a generous Kocher maneuver so as to free up the distal duodenal bulb and the entire descending portion of the duodenum, and to mobilize the bulb medially from its retroperitoneal attachments. Secondly, a horizontal incision is made across the pylorus. The incision should extend 2 to 2.5 cm on both gastric and duodenal sides of the pylorus. Traction sutures are then placed through the serosa on the pylorus, superior and inferior to the horizontal incision.

B. Traction on these sutures converts the incision to a vertical one, which is then closed with interrupted sutures. Many surgeons use simple interrupted sutures.

C. Use of three or four Gambee stitches will better preserve the lumen. These sutures go full-thickness through the gastric wall into the gastric lumen, then into the gastric mucosa at the edge and out at the gastric muscularis, then into the duodenal muscularis and through the duodenal mucosa to the duodenal lumen, and then out through the full thickness of the duodenum, from lumen to serosa. The function of the stitch is to bring the two walls together while inverting the mucosa, so as to keep the mucosa out of the way, and allow muscle-to-muscle approximation.

D. This figure shows the insertion of three of the Gambee sutures.

E. This figure shows the completed pyloroplasty. Some surgeons have advocated placement of a tab of omentum over the pyloroplasty, but since this maneuver has infrequently led to scarring and torsion of the pylorus so as to produce obstruction, I avoid it.

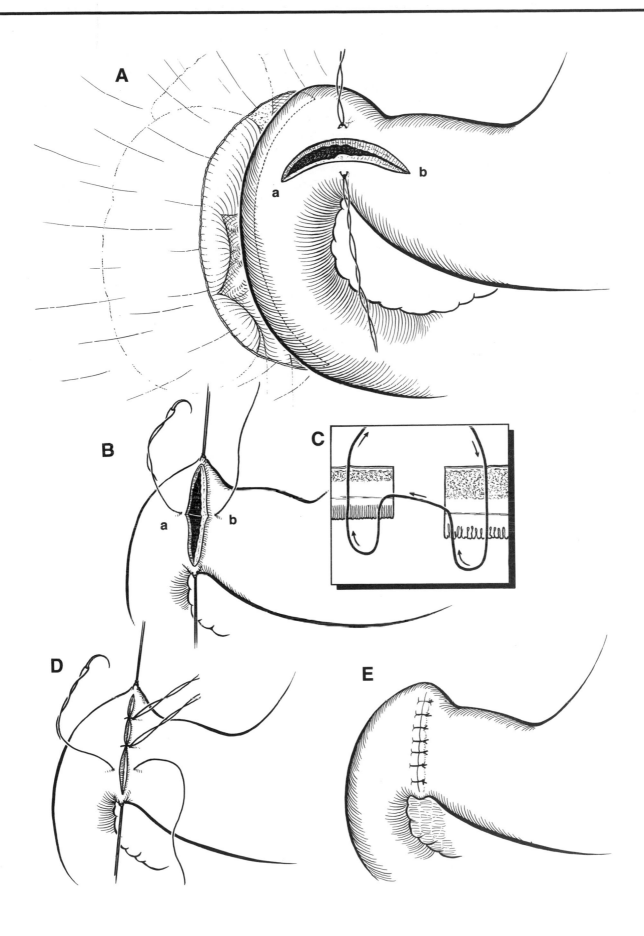

An alternative technique for pyloroplasty is the Finney method, which is actually a gastroduodenostomy created between the distal stomach and the proximal duodenum.

FIG 13–2

A. After a decision has been made to provide gastric drainage by means of a Finney pyloroplasty, the first step is to do a generous Kocher maneuver, so as to free up the lateral border of the first and second parts of the duodenum. The descending limb of the duodenum is then moved medially so as to be parallel to the distal greater curvature of the stomach, and a row of interrupted 4-0 polyglactin (Vicryl) sutures is placed between the stomach and duodenum.

B. After the posterior row of serosal sutures is completed, a full-thickness incision is made on both sides (that is, gastric and duodenal) of the suture line. The size of the anastomosis (usually 3 to 4 cm) depends upon the length of the suture line, that is, the distance between *b* and *c* in this diagram. The two parallel incisions (dotted lines) into the stomach and duodenum are then connected above the superior end of the suture line (marked *b*) with a curved continuation of the incision, the apex of which is marked as *a*.

C. The posterior suture line of the full-thickness closure is initiated at point *b* using a continuous running locking 4-0 Vicryl suture carried from *b* towards *c*. At the inferior aspect of the gastroduodenostomy, the suture is brought out through the wall of the stomach, and then continued anteriorly as a Connell suture.

D. This Connell suture line is then carried superiorly along the length of the gastroduodenostomy, so as to provide a full-thickness, inverting suture line.

E. The anterior continuous Connell suture line is then reinforced with a row of interrupted 4-0 polyglactin sutures. When the anastomosis is completed, there should be a wide-open aperture between distal stomach and proximal duodenum.

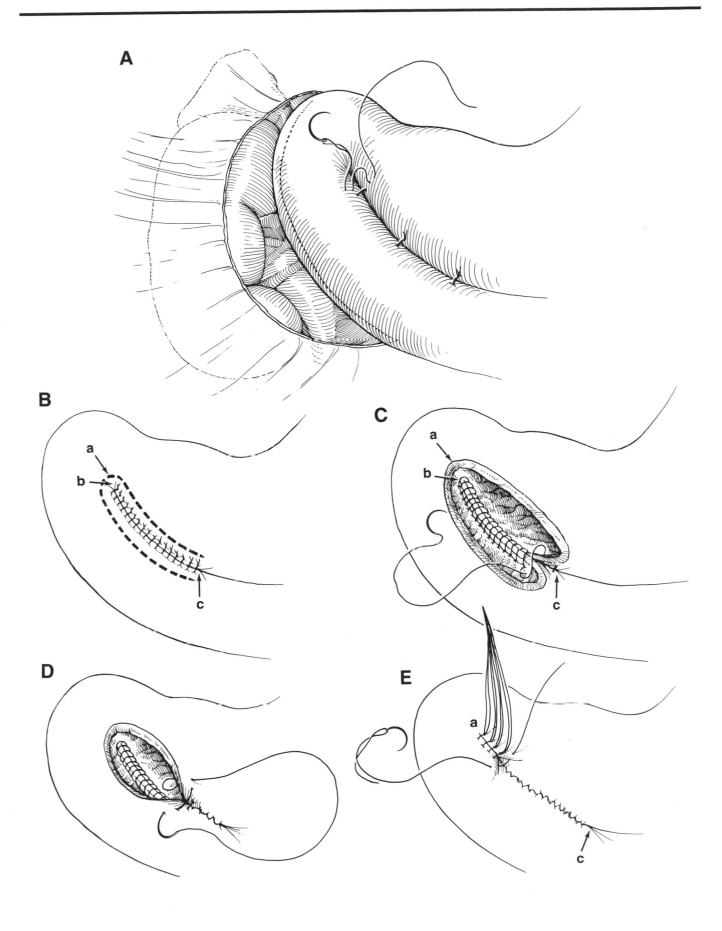

Antrectomy
and Truncal Vagotomy

14

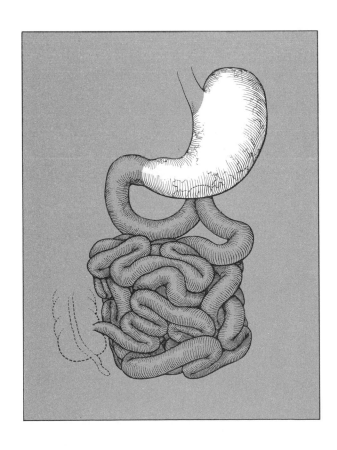

After Dragstedt introduced truncal vagotomy and drainage for treatment of duodenal ulcer, surgeons realized that success of operative procedures was proportional to the degree of reduction of gastric acidity. In treatment of duodenal ulcer disease, subtotal gastrectomy achieved success in reducing acid secretion by removing the antral gastrin mechanism and by the excision of variable amounts of the gastric fundus, which removed a part of the mass of parietal cells, thereby diminishing the size of the acid factory.

Soon after introduction of vagotomy, several surgeons seized upon the idea of combining the acid-reducing effects of vagotomy with those of antrectomy, and by the mid-1950s, surgeons in Boston, New York, and Nashville had large series of patients in whom they achieved great success in treating duodenal ulcer by means of truncal vagotomy and antrectomy. When gastric resection was combined with truncal vagotomy, the superiority of the Billroth II anastomosis noted after subtotal gastrectomy alone (especially in reports from the Mayo Clinic) was lost, and most surgeons utilized the gastroduodenostomy (which has the theoretical advantage of retaining normal duodenal mechanisms for the inhibition of gastric acid secretion).

Although most surgeons limit truncal vagotomy and antrectomy to patients with intractable, or scarred, or perforated, or bleeding, or obstructed duodenal ulcer, some surgeons have utilized the procedure in patients with gastric ulcer, particularly those located near the pyloric channel, especially in patients who have high acid output associated with distal gastric ulcers. We have only rarely combined vagotomy with distal gastric resection for gastric ulcer disease. In my opinion, probably the only indication would be in a patient who had both a pyloric ulcer and high acid output.

FIG 14–1

A. This figure shows the scarred anterior surface of the duodenal bulb.

B. When distal gastric resection for duodenal ulcer disease is combined with vagotomy, the degree of acid reduction is greater than that achieved with any other operative procedure except total gastrectomy. Removal of more than 50% of the stomach had been blamed for deleterious nutritional consequences after gastrectomy, so that most surgeons who combined resection with truncal vagotomy found they could excise simply the antrum, leaving 50% to 60% of the proximal stomach, and still get good (in fact, just about the best) postoperative cure rates. After opening the abdomen and mobilizing the stomach and confirming the ulcer, truncal vagotomy is carried out as illustrated (Chapter 11). The line of division of the stomach should be proximal to the antrofundic junction, shown in the illustration as an undulating dotted line. For years, I practiced a technique for identifying the antrum by performing a generous gastrotomy, drying out all gastric secretions within the stomach, administering pentagastrin intravenously and laying strips of pH paper transversely across the antrofundic junction. In general, the antrum is smaller in patients with high acid output and relatively larger in patients with low acid output. In nearly every patient with duodenal ulcer disease, we found that excision along a line drawn from the lesser curvature about 1 to 1.5 cm proximal to the incisura angularis and angling toward the greater curvature at an angle of about 40 degrees to the vertical (shown in the illustration as the *heavy dotted line*) would completely excise antral mucosa. Since in this operation any residual antral mucosa would be in permanent continuity with acid-secreting fundic mucosa, the need to excise every single bit of fundic mucosa is not critical.

C. Division of the stomach followed by closure of the lesser curvature and the gastroduodenostomy are all carried out as illustrated in Chapter 7. The completed truncal vagotomy and antrectomy and gastroduodenostomy are shown here. If a gastrojejunostomy is chosen, the anastomosis is carried out as illustrated in Chapter 9.

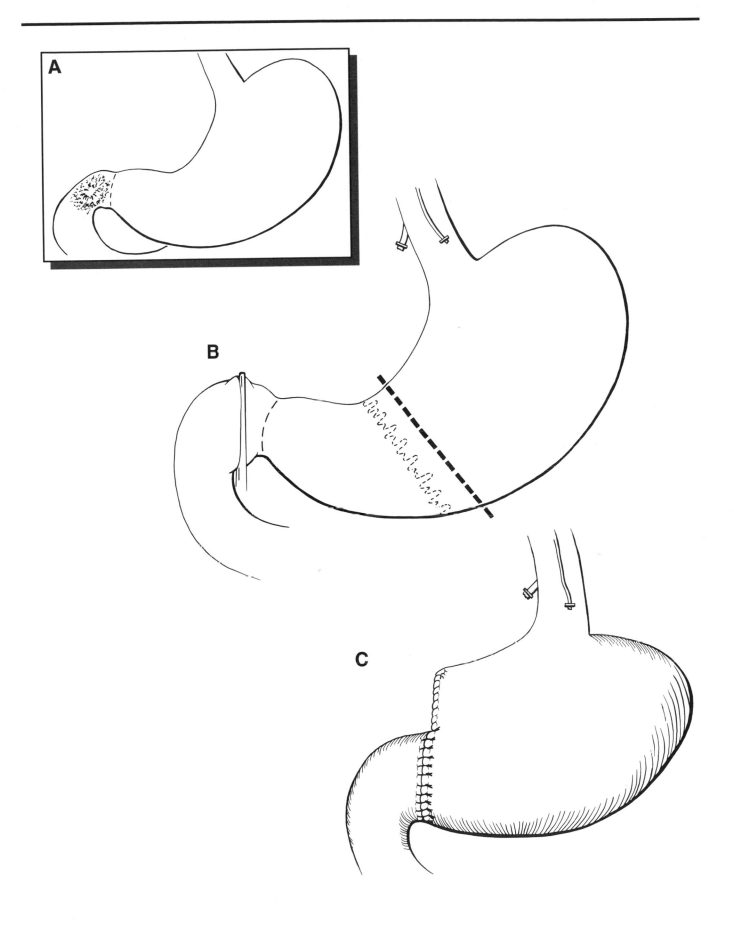

A

B

C

Antrectomy and Truncal Vagotomy

Selective Total Gastric Vagotomy Plus Drainage

15

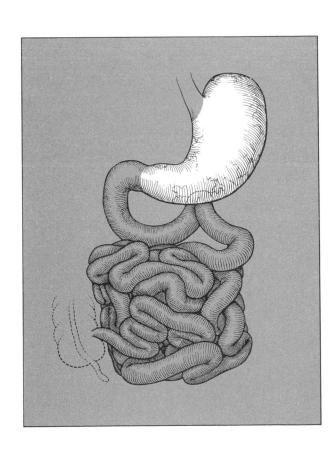

Selective total gastric vagotomy plus drainage for the treatment of peptic ulcer disease was introduced as a means of improving the completeness of vagotomy while at the same time preserving hepatic and celiac branches of the vagi. The technique is similar to that of selective proximal vagotomy (see Chapter 16) except that the denervation is carried distally all the way to the pylorus, thereby denervating the antral musculature. Antral denervation greatly impedes gastric emptying so that a drainage procedure (either pyloroplasty or gastrojejunostomy) is required. The technique of selective proximal vagotomy with preservation of the antral innervation does not require a drainage procedure and in most areas selective proximal vagotomy has displaced selective total gastric vagotomy. Long experience with total gastric vagotomy for duodenal ulcer by Amdrup and colleagues in Aarhus, Denmark, however, has yielded very good results. The operation is certainly uncommon.

FIG 15–1

A. This figure shows a completed total gastric vagotomy with division of the anterior and posterior leaves of the gastrohepatic ligament and their contained nerves and blood vessels. This procedure is identical to selective proximal vagotomy (see Chapter 16), except that the dissection is carried all the way from the *pylorus* to the esophageal hiatus. At the beginning of the procedure, the vagal trunks are identified (see Chapter 11) and tagged with a heavy silk suture so as to allow for easy identification and to prevent inadvertent division of the trunks. This shows the *(dotted)* line of the pyloroplasty incision and the two stay sutures.

B. A Heineke-Mikulicz pyloroplasty is then performed as previously illustrated (see Fig 13–1). This figure shows the completed procedure of total gastric vagotomy and pyloroplasty.

C. An alternative technique is to complete the total gastric vagotomy and then provide drainage with a gastrojejunostomy.

D. The gastrojejunostomy can be created either in front of or behind the transverse colon. Illustrated here is an anterior gastrojejunostomy, as previously described (see Chapter 12).

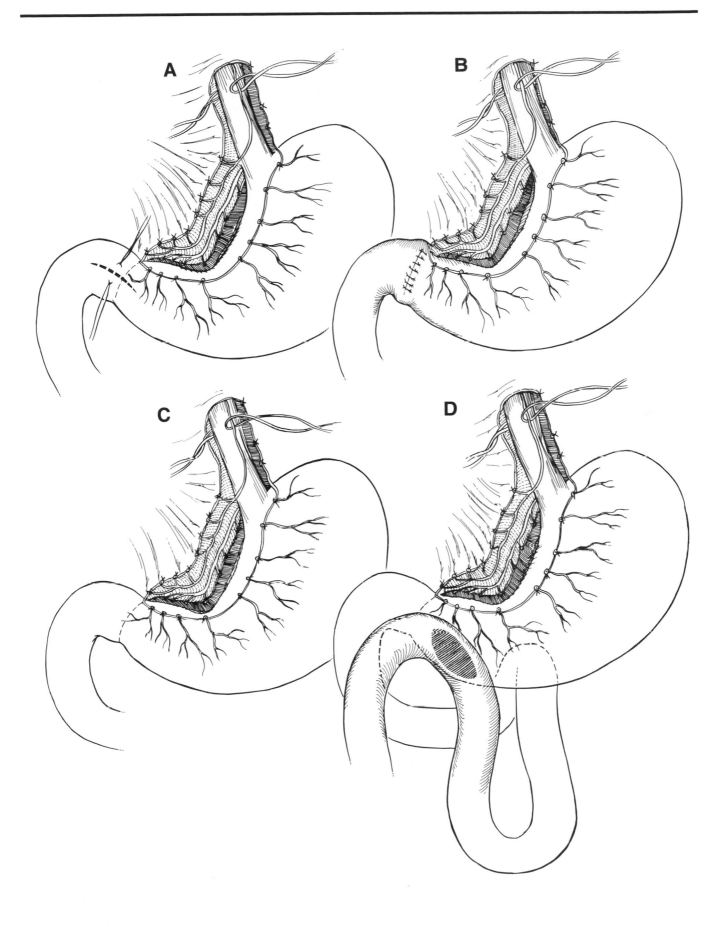

Selective Proximal Vagotomy*

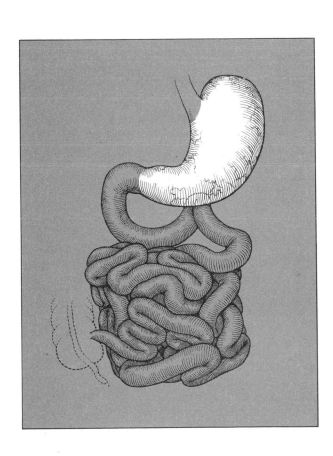

*Also called highly selective vagotomy, supraselective vagotomy, proximal gastric vagotomy, and parietal cell vagotomy, among other terms.

Selective proximal vagotomy, also called highly selective vagotomy, supraselective vagotomy, proximal gastric vagotomy, and parietal cell vagotomy, is the long-awaited ideal physiologic procedure for reduction of gastric acid. It achieves denervation of the parietal cell mass while preserving innervation to the antral smooth muscle, the pump that empties the stomach. Since the lumen of the gut is not opened, the procedure is extraordinarily safe (and since the innervation of the rest of the abdominal viscera is preserved, as is the integrity of the pylorus, dumping and diarrhea are nearly eradicated). Some questions of technical judgment remain: for example, how far distally and proximally to carry the denervation. We now agree that the proximal denervation should go all the way to the diaphragmatic hiatus for the esophagus, but the distal extent of denervation is still unsettled. The choice is important because if denervation is carried too far distally, the antrum is denervated and gastric stasis results (a condition that led Fritz Holle to add submucosal anterior pylorectomy to his operation). If distal denervation is insufficient, the innervation of distal fundic parietal cells remains intact and acid production may remain high. We address the problem arbitrarily. We choose a spot 7 cm from the pylorus on the lesser curvature and inspect the crow's foot anatomy of the nerve of Latarjet as it crosses onto the antrum. Those fibers that go proximalward toward the fundus, we divide.

Some surgeons, Holle for instance, meticulously divide only the nerve fibers to the fundus, preserving vascular connections. Most surgeons, however, serially divide the entire gastrohepatic ligament, first the anterior leaf and then the posterior leaf, and in the process divide all neural and all vascular connections of the lesser curvature, from the diaphragm to the incisura angularis. Technique must be meticulous. Often, the ties on the stomach wall may be loosened by repeated rubbing contact during the operation and vessels may bleed. Suture ligatures are helpful to handle this bleeding, and in fact, some surgeons use suture ligatures *primarily* on the gastric side of the divided gastrohepatic ligament in order to prevent bleeding. Care should be taken to avoid hematomas; they obscure the view and make dissection difficult. Visualization of the nerve of Latarjet, as it descends in the gastrohepatic ligament, greatly facilitates the entire operation.

We find it helpful to maintain straight distal traction on the greater curvature of the stomach by having an assistant grasp the greater curvature over an inlying nasogastric tube and hold the stomach tautly distal with two hands around a laparotomy sponge placed around the stomach. In the course of dissection of the posterior leaf of the gastrohepatic ligament along the lesser curvature, a vein retractor lifting the lesser curvature may facilitate exposure.

There is a definite learning curve for this procedure and the surgeon should meticulously measure gastric acid output in his first five to ten patients until he can be sure that he is achieving good reduction of acid output. You do get better and faster. My first four cases averaged 4 hours each. My last 10 cases averaged 2 hours, with a few thin patients undergoing the operation in 70 to 80 minutes.

FIG 16–1

A. We use a midline incision from the xiphoid to below the umbilicus.

B. Exposure is facilitated by use of a Goligher sternal retractor (or any upper hand retractor). We place a Finochietto retractor for lateral exposure and a Weinberg retractor for exposure of the interabdominal esophagus. Use of the Weinberg retractor makes division of the triangular ligament of the liver unnecessary for retraction of the left lobe of the liver. This figure shows the excellent exposure secured by means of the Finochietto and Weinberg retractors.

C. To mobilize the esophagus, the operator passes his hand around the esophagus (easily identified by the inlying nasogastric tube). The esophagus is lifted anteriorly and the phrenoesophageal ligament behind the esophagus is placed under pressure using the long finger.

D. The phrenoesophageal ligament posterior to the esophagus is broken through by blunt dissection and the aperture is enlarged proximalward and distalward by means of blunt dissection.

E. A medium Penrose drain is then placed around the esophagus and placed on tension to facilitate mobilization of the esophagus. The phrenoesophageal ligament is completely divided posteriorly from the stomach to the diaphragm.

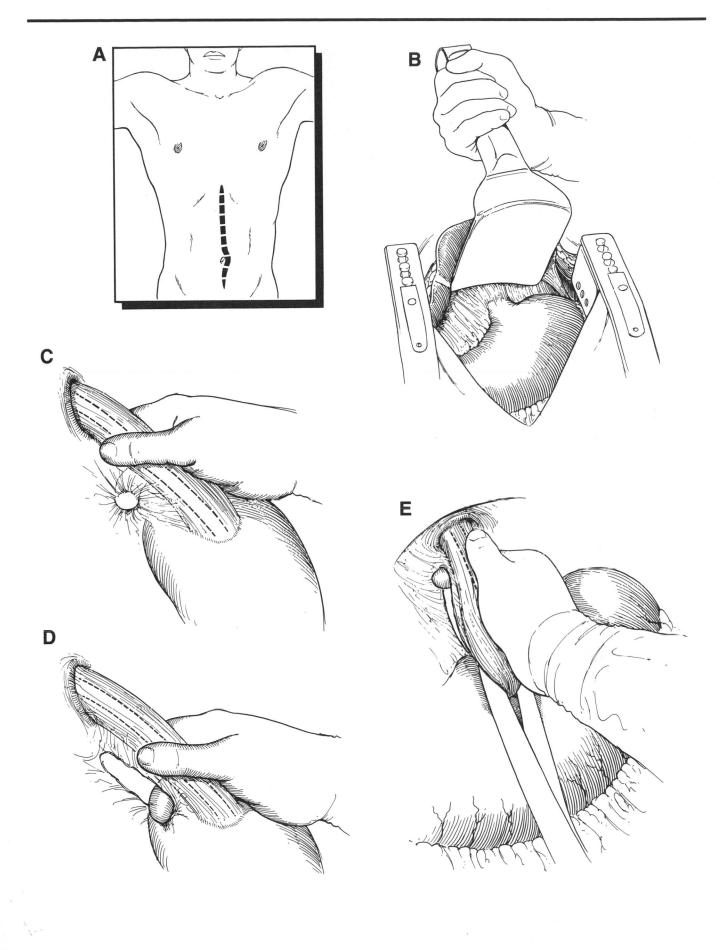

F. Blunt dissection is carried around laterally and anteriorly so as to obliterate all of the phrenoesophageal ligament and skeletonize the esophagus. With tension on the esophagus by means of the Penrose drain, the small anterior and the large posterior vagal trunks are easily palpated. The anterior vagus is usually located at about the 1 o'clock position (with the xiphoid at 12 o'clock) and the posterior vagus is at about 6:30 or 7 o'clock.

G. We place long, heavy silk sutures around the anterior and posterior vagi to facilitate their identification during the operation. The descending nerves of Latarjet will be serially freed from their attachments to the fundus, and as the dissection proceeds proximally, it is possible to divide vagal trunks accidentally. This accident, of course, would vitiate the entire operation. Tags on the main vagal trunks will serve to protect against that accident.

H. The Weinberg retractor is removed and attention directed to the distal stomach. Traction is placed on the greater curvature, as described above, and a point on the lesser curvature about 7 cm proximal to the pylorus is selected and tagged with a suture.

I. After the suture tag is placed at 7 cm, the anatomy of the nerve of Latarjet is carefully inspected. The nerve breaks up into numerous branches (the crow's foot) as it passes onto the antrum. All branches of nerve fibers that course in a proximal direction (that is, back toward the fundus) are divided. As shown in these illustrations, the line of division of the gastrohepatic ligament begins at 7 cm on the lesser curvature. In the upper illustration, two branches of the nerve of Latarjet, distal to the line of division, are found to go in a proximal direction and they have been divided. In the lower illustration, one branch goes in a proximal direction and has been divided. Tension on the nerve of Latarjet with a nerve hook will facilitate identification of the smaller branches.

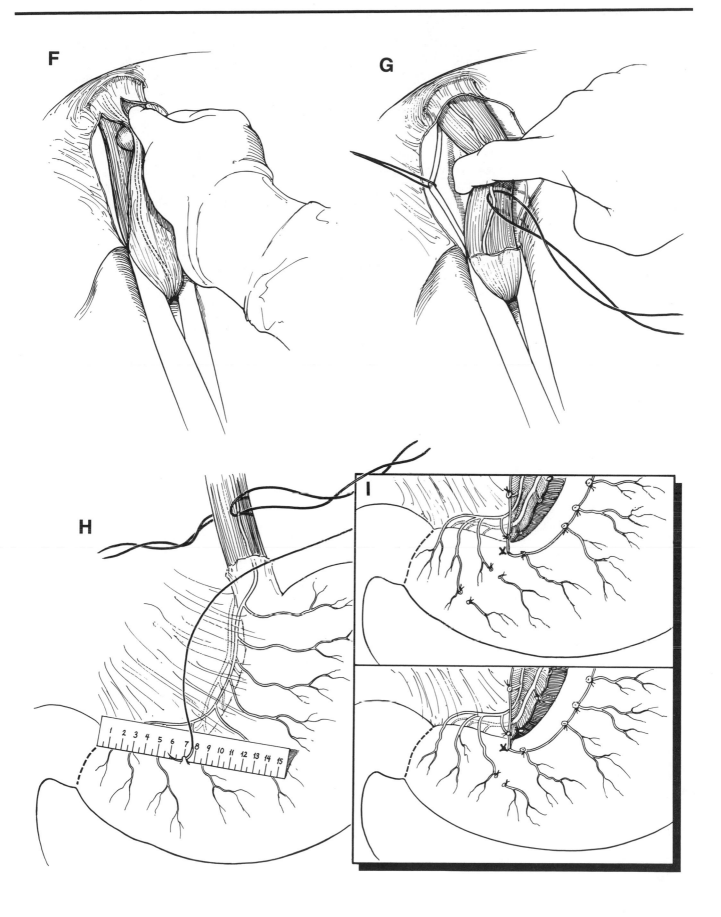

J. Exposure is facilitated by placing the nasogastric tube fully into the stomach along the lesser curvature all the way to the pylorus. The indwelling nasogastric tube can then be grasped by an assistant using a sponge wrapped around the tube within the greater curvature, applying straight distal (inferior) traction. This traction facilitates exposure of the structures within the gastrohepatic omentum and facilitates ligation of the neurovascular bundles coming from the gastrohepatic omentum to the lesser curvature of the stomach.

K. The serial division of the anterior leaf of the gastrohepatic omentum is carried out by placing a clamp underneath nerve, artery, and vein, opening the clamp so as to secure sufficient space so that two ligatures may be placed with a small intervening cuff of tissue. One suture (we use either 3-0 silk or 4-0 polyglactin [Vicryl]) is pulled through and then another suture is pulled through.

L. The two sutures are separated and tied. As noted elsewhere, it is important to secure as much distance as possible between the two ligatures so as to retain a cuff of tissue to mitigate against slippage of the vessel back through the ligature. During the course of dissection this often happens to vessels on the stomach, and the best response is a transfixion ligature to suture-ligate the offending vessel.

M. After ligating the branches of the nerve of Latarjet (along with arterial and venous branches), the clamp is replaced underneath the ligated tissue, which is then divided.

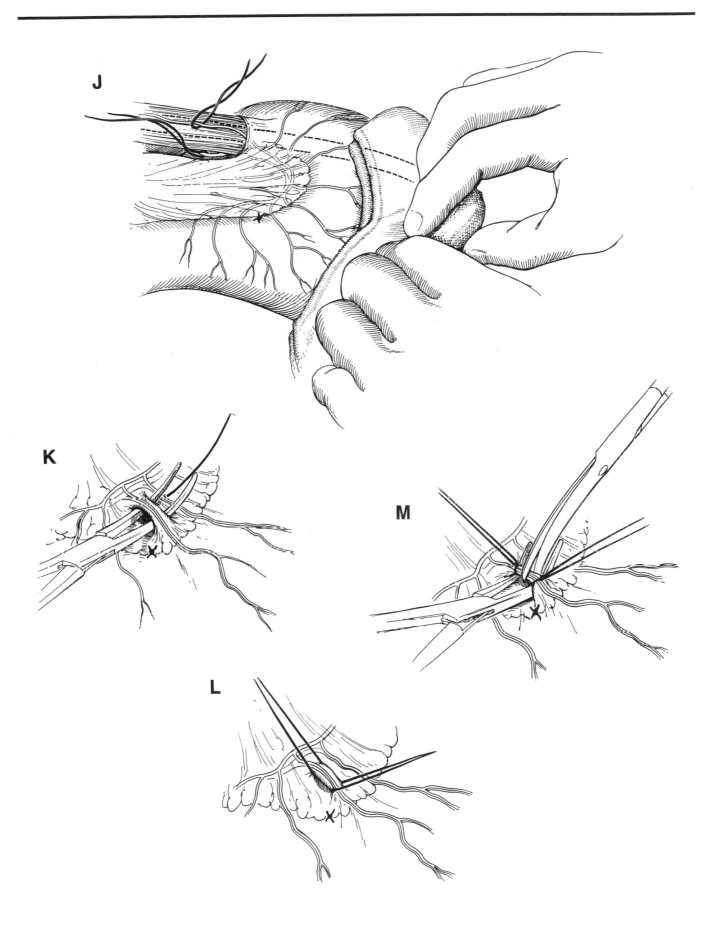

N. This illustration of a cross section of the junction of the gastrohepatic ligament with lesser curvature shows the placement of the anterior *(1)* and posterior *(2)* nerves of Laterjet, along with the marginal artery *(3)* and vein *(4)*.

O. The entire anterior leaf of the gastrohepatic ligament is divided serially between ligatures, from the incisura to the esophageal hiatus. Once this is done, there is usually an intermediate layer of neurovascular structures that must be ligated and divided before going entirely through the gastrohepatic ligament into the lesser omental bursa. At this point, exposure is often facilitated by lifting the lesser curvature of the stomach with a vein retractor, as shown here. The procedure is repeated on the posterior leaf. At the end of the dissection, the entire lesser curvature from the incisura angularis to the esophagus is freed of all neurovascular attachments.

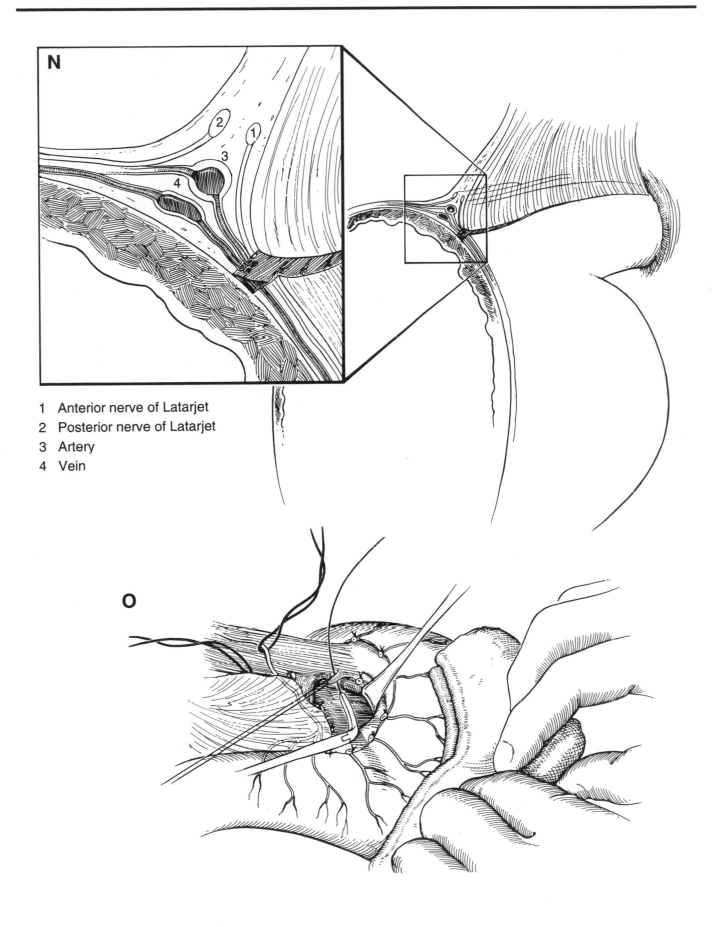

1 Anterior nerve of Latarjet
2 Posterior nerve of Latarjet
3 Artery
4 Vein

P. This shows the completed dissection. We spend some time looking for any bleeders or any sutures that may have been brushed off. At the finish, we reperitonealize the lesser curvature by bringing together the edges of the serosa with a running suture so as to cover the bare exposed area of the lesser curvature. We do this to prevent adhesions. Some maintain that the maneuver diminishes resprouting of nerve fibers.

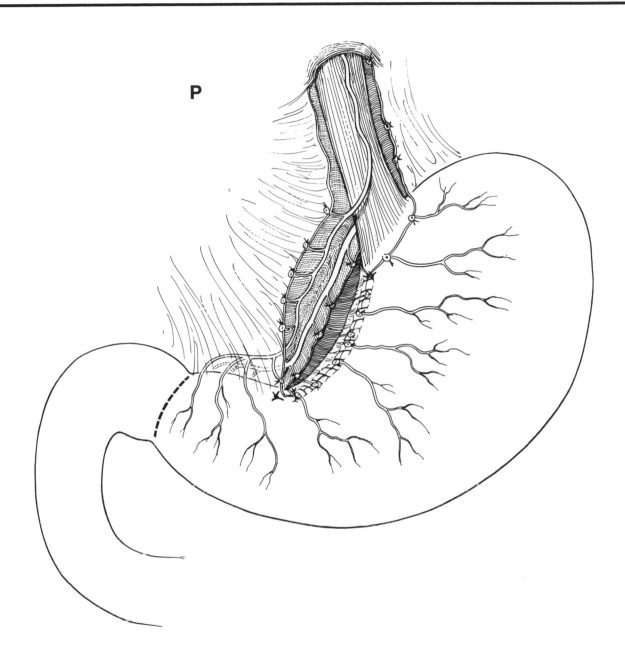

P

Pyloroplasty for Bleeding Duodenal Ulcer Using the U-Stitch

17

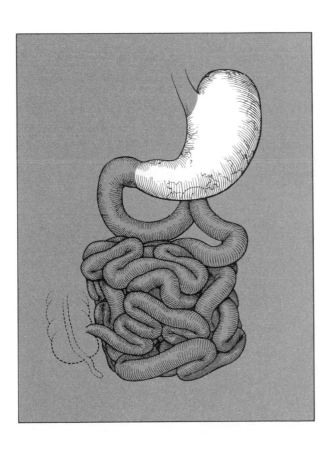

The management of bleeding duodenal ulcer by vagotomy, pyloroplasty and suture ligation of the bleeding ulcer base brought about great improvement in mortality, especially among older patients. The method was not foolproof, however, and the incidence of rebleeding after ligation of the ulcer was troublesomely high. The usual technique for ligation was to put a deep suture in the superior and in the inferior aspect of the ulcer crater thereby transfixing, presumably, the gastroduodenal artery. Berne and Rosoff (*Ann Surg* 1969;169:141) suggested that the rebleeding might be from a collateral anastomosis from the transverse pancreatic artery into the side of the gastroduodenal artery (see **Fig 1–1, B,** p. 5). They suggested that the potential bad result of such a collateral linkage could be averted by placement of a suture (which they called a U-stitch) to occlude the collateral. Application of this technique has diminished the incidence of post–suture ligation rebleeding.

FIG 17–1

A. The first step is to perform a Kocher maneuver, followed by a horizontal pyloroplasty incision.

B. Placement of traction sutures in the midportion of the superior and inferior limbs of the horizontal incision affords exposure of the bleeding ulcer. We use 2-0 silk for the U suture, which is placed as illustrated.

C. After the U-stitch is tied, a simple suture is taken above and below the ulcer crater so as to ligate the gastroduodenal artery.

D. The pyloroplasty is closed (see **Fig 13–1**, p. 85) and a truncal vagotomy performed (see Chapter 11).

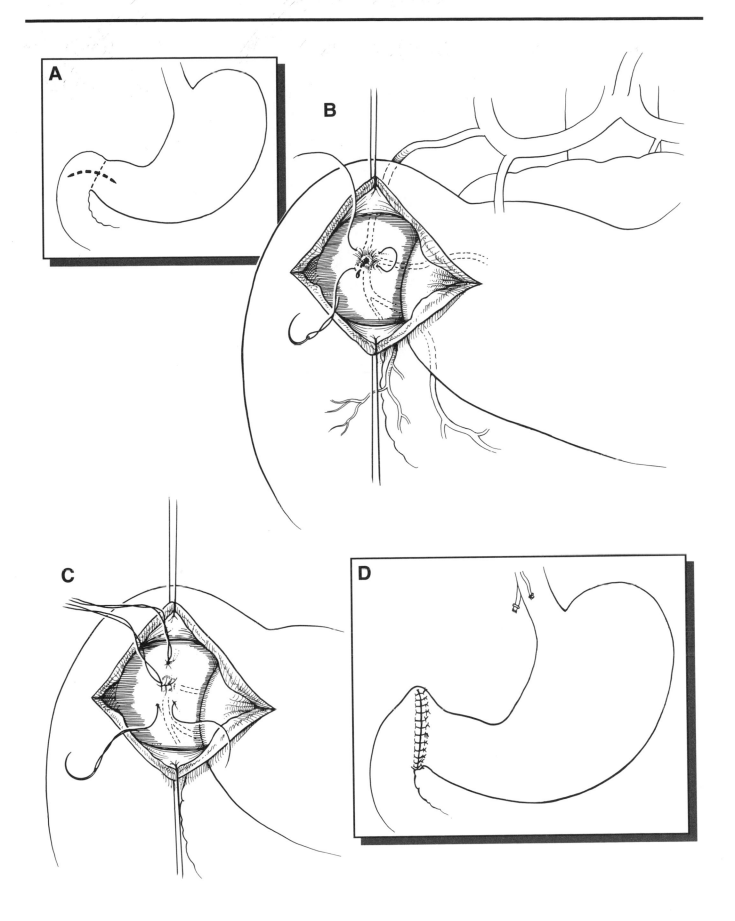

18

Perforation of Duodenal Ulcer: Treatment by Simple Closure or by Closure Plus Acid-Reducing Operation

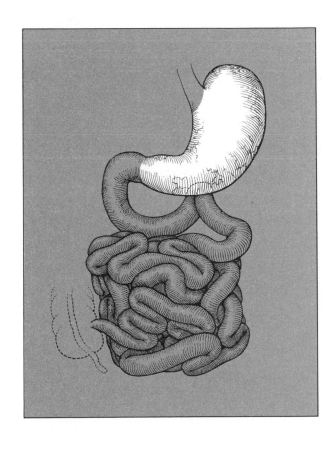

Perforation of a duodenal ulcer is a classic indication for operation. Perforating ulcers are usually located in the anterior wall of the duodenal bulb and the perforations classically occur suddenly, usually converting someone in good health to serious illness in a matter of minutes. The symptoms and physical findings are usually dramatic and in about 70% of cases the suspected diagnosis can be confirmed on upright chest x-ray by demonstration of free subdiaphragmatic intraperitoneal air. Duodenal ulcers may also perforate insidiously in chronically ill patients, some of whom have diseases of the central nervous system that render them comatose. In such instances, the diagnosis of ulcer perforation often requires a high degree of suspicion and the physician should think of perforation when asked to see any obtunded patient who has developed ileus suddenly. Free intraperitoneal air can be demonstrated in patients who cannot sit up by taking an x-ray film in the left lateral decubitus position.

Therapeutic options in patients with perforated ulcer are, first of all, operative or nonoperative. Although some success has been reported in the management of perforated ulcer by continuous nasogastric suction, most studies confirm the superiority of operation. Occasionally in a patient who appears days after perforation, the ulcer has already sealed, and the patient is in little distress. These patients, and patients who are clearly moribund from other causes, should not be operated upon.

When operating upon patients with perforation, the surgeon should decide whether or not to attempt an acid-reducing procedure as well. In general, we perform acid-reducing procedures on patients with a history of chronic duodenal ulcer disease, especially those with previous hemorrhage or perforation, or those who at operation show signs of incipient pyloric outlet obstruction and who are generally good operative risks. We do simple closures of perforations on patients in whom the perforation is an acute event without prior ulcer history, or in poor-risk patients in whom there is massive soilage and generalized peritonitis or in patients who are poor operative risks for any reason. In patients with an acute perforation and a pliable duodenum, simple closure may often be easily performed with a suture or two. Most patients, however, have thickened duodenal walls, walls that are often nearly cartilaginous in consistency, and the perforation may be large. Attempts to suture such perforations are often unsuccessful; sutures pull out or the tissue is too rigid to be approximated. This problem is managed by bringing up a tab of omentum and suturing it in place over the perforation.

FIG 18–1

A. Size and location of perforations vary. They may be pinpoint or large and indurated. Perforations of postbulbar ulcers are rare. If great contamination exists, perforations should be sealed by pressure with a sponge and the abdominal cavity cleansed. The duodenum, stomach, and adjacent gastrocolic and gastrohepatic ligaments are often edematous.
B. Large perforations with indurated edges are almost always best closed by bringing up a tab of omentum, a technique devised by Roscoe Graham of Toronto.
C. The sutures are tied with moderate tension, taking care to avoid strangulation of the omental patch. This technique, so-called Graham's closure, is usually highly successful. It does not, of course, affect the ulcer diathesis and the patient postoperatively is subject to the same vicissitudes of duodenal ulcer disease as before.
D. The options available for treatment of perforated duodenal ulcer by closure of the perforation plus a simultaneous acid-reducing procedure are excision of the anterior perforated ulcer and pyloroplasty and truncal vagotomy, or antrectomy plus vagotomy with excision of ulcer, or Graham's closure of ulcer plus selective proximal vagotomy. On occasion, in patients with badly distorted duodenal bulbs, we have used simple closure with a Graham's patch plus truncal vagotomy and gastroenterostomy. In performing truncal vagotomy plus pyloroplasty, the ulcer and surrounding zone of induration are excised with a transverse incision that goes across the pylorus, as shown here. This method, of course, is not applicable if the perforation is huge, or if the zone of induration encompasses the whole duodenal bulb.
E. The horizontal incision is then converted to a vertical wound and closed vertically in the Heineke-Mikulicz fashion (see Chapter 13).
F. The completed procedure of ulcer excision, Heineke-Mikulicz pyloroplasty and truncal vagotomy is shown here.

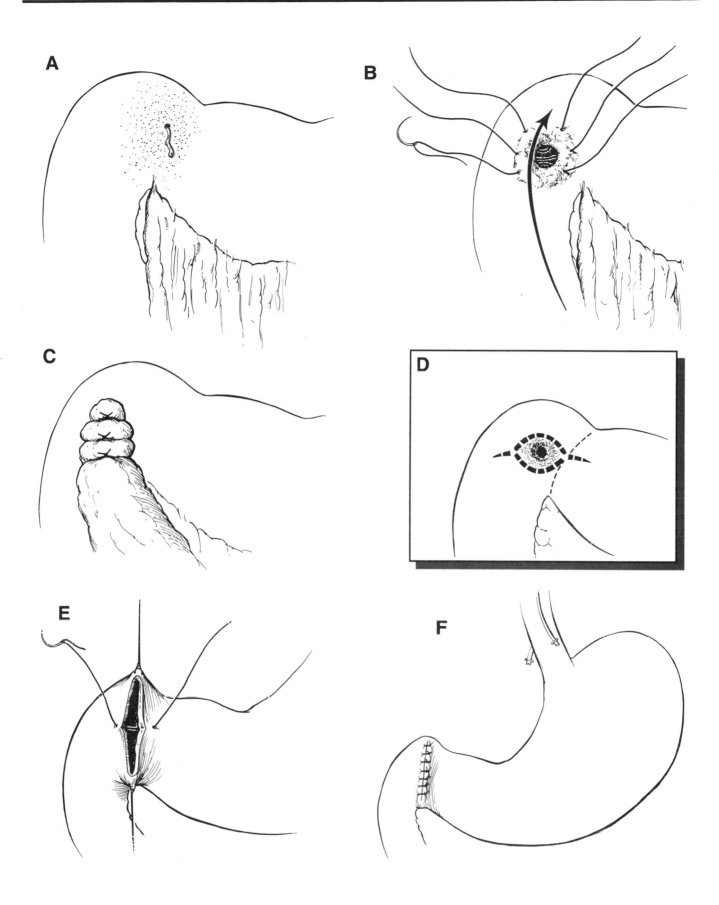

G.   Another means of managing a perforated duodenal ulcer and achieving acid reduction is to resect the distal stomach and proximal duodenum and to do a truncal vagotomy. This figure shows planned lines of resection for a hemigastrectomy. Excision of the proximal duodenum must be done with care so as to allow sufficient length to carry out a Billroth I anastomosis. The feasibility of this method depends entirely upon the degree of duodenal distortion and whether or not the duodenum can be mobilized from the pancreas. I do not favor this method because of difficulty in anastomosing the indurated duodenum to the stomach. It is popular in some centers.

H.   This shows the completed operation of antrectomy, vagotomy, and Billroth I gastroduodenostomy. Dissection of the distal stomach and gastroduodenostomy is carried out as illustrated in Chapter 7. Truncal vagotomy is carried out as illustrated in Chapter 11.

I.   Several recent articles have provided evidence that simple closure of the perforation plus selective proximal vagotomy may give good results. This figure illustrates the completed procedure with a Graham closure (see **B** and **C**) and a selective proximal vagotomy (see Chapter 16).

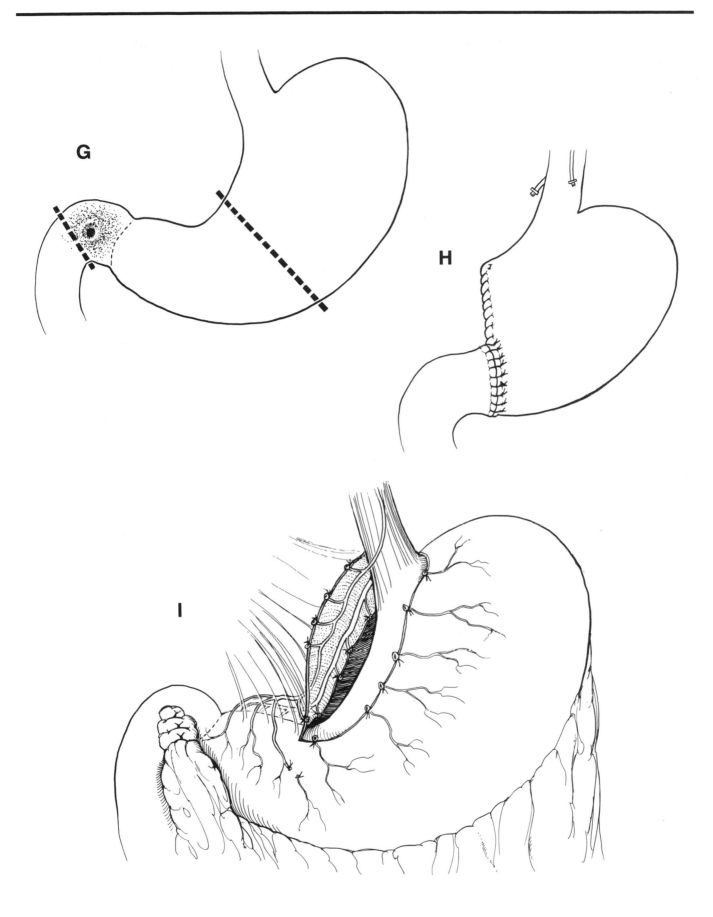

J. In patients with a badly scarred duodenum, we have on occasion performed a Graham closure plus truncal vagotomy plus anterior gastrojejunostomy. The Graham closure is carried out as in **B** and **C** above, the truncal vagotomy is carried out as in Chapter 11, and the anterior gastrojejunostomy is carried out as in Chapter 12.

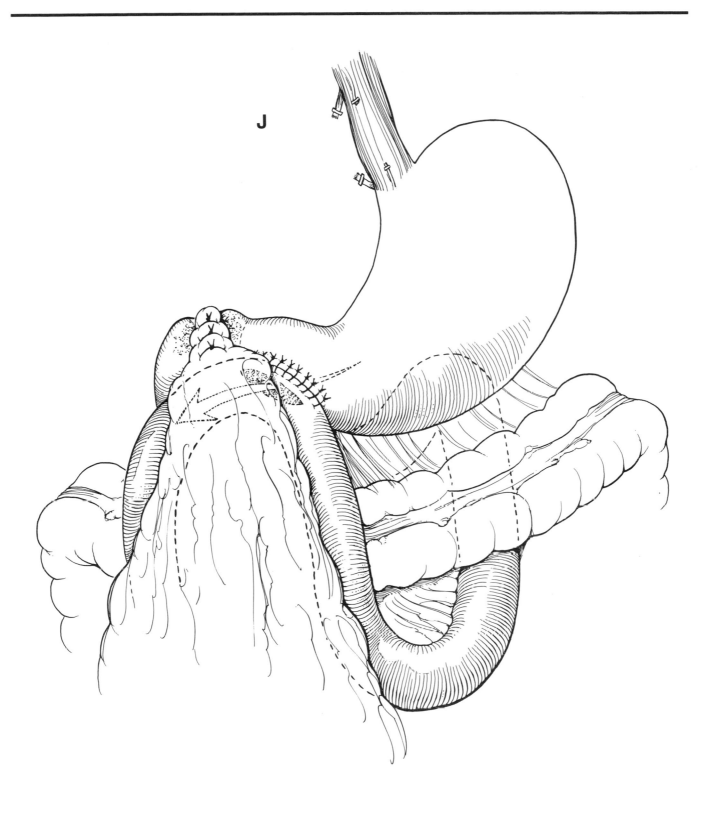

J

Procedures for Benign Gastric Outlet Obstruction

Procedures for Benign Gastric Outlet Obstruction

19

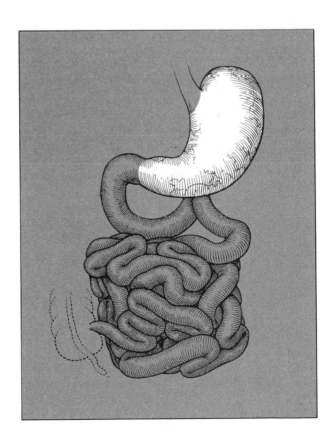

19

121

Pyloric obstruction, along with hemorrhage and perforation, constitute three anatomic complications of peptic ulcer disease that may require operative treatment (intractibility or failure of conservative therapy is the fourth indication). Pyloric obstruction occurs as a consequence of scarring that is incident to repeated cycles of remissions and exacerbations of peptic ulcer in the pyloric region. The responsible ulcer is usually located in the first part of the duodenum, but the scarring occurs just at the pylorus, and with each episode of healing contraction of the scar increases until ultimately the pyloric outlet is narrowed so as to create obstruction, first to solid food and then to passage of liquid. Experienced surgeons and gastroenterologists know that although one might, in theory, expect gastric outlet obstruction to produce dramatic symptoms, the gradual narrowing of the pyloric outlet is often compensated by progressive thickening of the muscular coat causing increased force of gastric contraction and later by progressive gastric dilatation. By the time actual obstruction occurs, the symptoms are often quite insidious. Patients may, of course, present with violent emesis and severe electrolyte derangement (classically a hypokalemic, hypochloremic alkalosis), but usually the patient comes in with mild overflow vomiting, usually of a brackish, watery fluid. The stomach may be hugely dilated and the walls coated with layers of retained food. The degree of obstruction may be estimated by upper GI barium x-ray, but the best way of estimation is perform endoscopy and visualize the pylorus. We find that if we cannot pass an adult endoscope into the duodenum significant obstruction exists and the patient will almost always require operation. Once this degree of obstruction is present, we believe it is important to proceed with operation since the chance of spontaneous remission is slim to nonexistent. We formerly used the saline load test to estimate degree of obstruction (as well as prognosis); endoscopy is better.

The stomach should be thoroughly decompressed prior to operation; this may take days of vigorous irrigation to remove the layers of food plastered to the gastric wall. We take a large Ewald tube and irrigate for 20 minutes (or as long as we and the patient can stand it) three times a day. Failure of gastric emptying is the most common complication after operation for pyloric outlet obstruction, and we believe that the period of waiting for return of gastric function can be decreased by 2 or 3 days of preoperative nasogastric suction, after careful emptying of all gastric content, so as to allow the muscle wall of the stomach to regain tone. Nonetheless, patient and family must be warned preoperatively that postoperative resumption of gastric emptying may be slow.

The operative approaches include vagotomy, usually truncal vagotomy as shown here, coupled with either resection or drainage. I have recently used selective proximal vagotomy with drainage to treat this condition.

FIG 19–1

A. This figure shows the pyloric stenosis and the dilated, hypertrophied stomach. Truncal vagotomy is carried out (see Chapter 11) and the distal stomach is either drained or resected.

B. If we resect, we use antrectomy plus Billroth I reconstruction (see Chapter 14). The problem with this approach is that the duodenum is badly scarred and difficult to mobilize, and may present trouble in the surgeon's attempt to create an anastomosis. Occasionally it may be possible during the resection to excise the scarred duodenum and get beyond the narrowed segment, but this is unusual. For this reason, we do not favor resection and gastroduodenostomy except in the rare instance in which the site of obstruction is immediately prepyloric and the obstructed zone can be easily resected.

C. The simplest way, in my opinion, to provide drainage for an obstructed stomach after truncal vagotomy is to perform a gastroenterostomy. We usually use an anterior gastrojejunostomy (see Chapter 12), although the choice between an antecolic or a retrocolic anastomosis depends upon the preference of the surgeon. We always try to make a large (3 to 4 cm) stoma and to create the stoma in the distal stomach so as to facilitate drainage. Although it is commonly used, I do not believe that Heineke-Mikulicz pyloroplasty is a good alternative in patients with pyloric outlet obstruction. The pylorus and proximal duodenum are heavily scarred and pyloroplasty is apt to provide insufficient drainage, or to leak, or both.

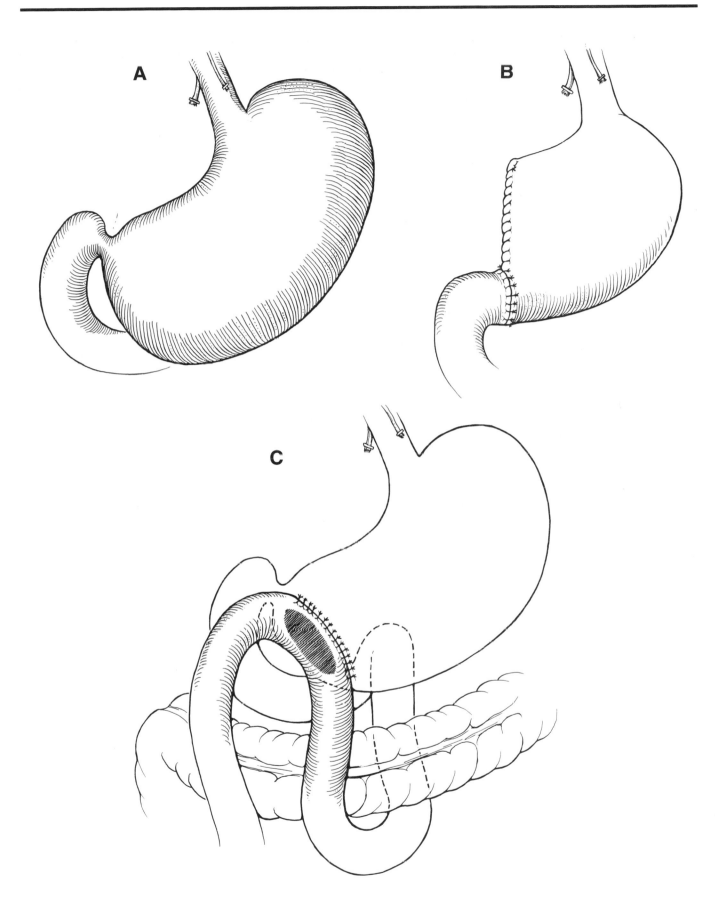

D. Because postoperative gastric stasis is a problem in patients with gastric outlet obstruction, we have on several occasions in the last few years performed a selective proximal vagotomy and drainage. This procedure allows denervation of the acid-secreting fundus with preservation of those vagal fibers that innervate the circular smooth muscle of the antrum, the pump that empties the stomach. The selective proximal vagotomy is carried out as depicted in Chapter 16.

E. After performing the proximal selective vagotomy, we assure gastric drainage by creating a gastroenterostomy. We have not yet treated sufficient numbers of patients by this technique to provide firm evidence that selective proximal vagotomy is superior to truncal vagotomy, but it is certainly our impression that the stomach empties sooner when antral innervation is preserved. Pyloric outlet obstruction is probably not amenable to treatment by selective proximal vagotomy plus pyloric dilatation. David Johnston and others reported initial success in patients with pyloric outlet obstruction who were treated by selective proximal vagotomy and intraoperative transgastric dilatation of the pyloric outlet. Later restenosis prevailed in most of these patients, however, and I believe the procedure has been generally abandoned. I believe that any use of selective proximal vagotomy in these patients should be accompanied by drainage.

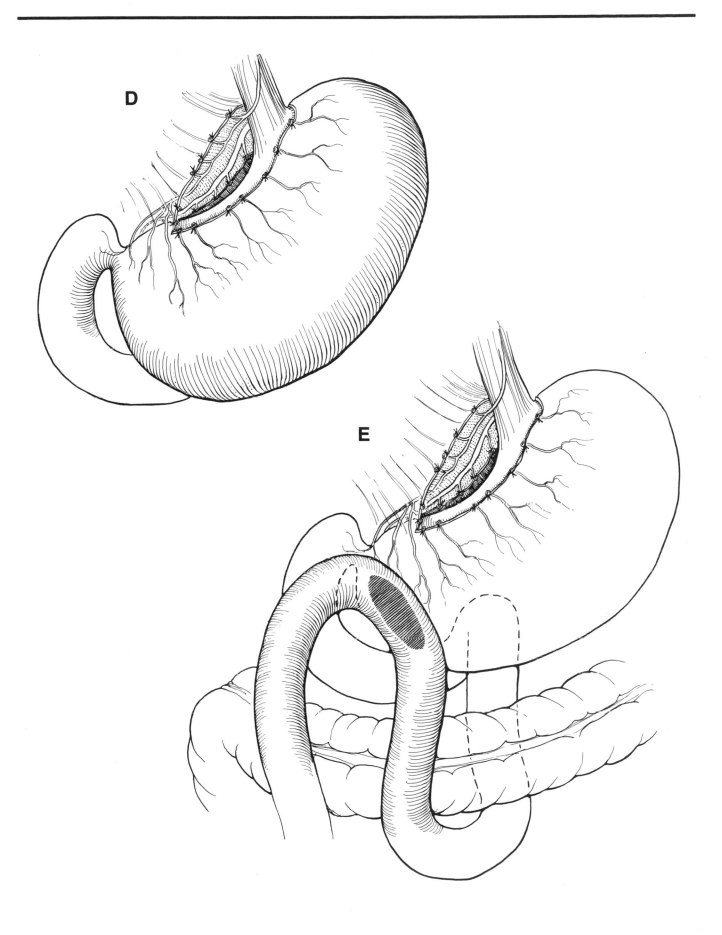

D

E

Perforation
of Gastric Ulcer

20

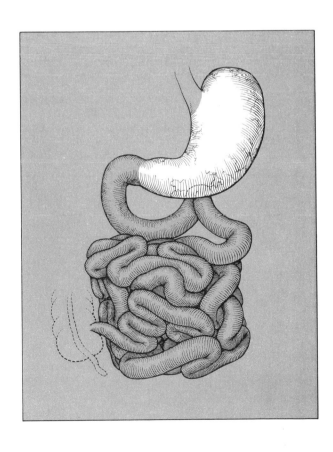

Chronic ulceration of the proximal stomach is unusual and perforations of proximal ulcers are fortunately rare. They are difficult to manage. First of all, the question of malignancy of the gastric ulcer must be settled. The technique for biopsy has been illustrated (see Chapter 7). If the ulcer is malignant, total gastrectomy should be considered (see Chapter 25). If excision of the ulcer appears inadvisable, simple closure may rarely be indicated (see **Fig 20–2,E**, p. 131). Most perforations are benign and since perforations of proximal gastric ulcers are often associated with bleeding, simple closure is usually not a good option. The two common choices for dealing with perforated proximal gastric ulcers are local excision and gastric resection. Patients are often old, fragile, and in poor condition; for this reason we often choose a free-hand excision of the ulcer with a closure that is tailored to the site of the ulcer. If the perforation is near the cardia, care must be taken so as not to compromise the opening of the esophagus into the stomach. For this reason, insertion of a no. 40 F Maloney dilator through the esophagus into the stomach will serve to protect the lumen.

FIG 20–1

A. Areas of perforation should be excised so as to get rid of the indurated and necrotic tissue. The exact method will, of course, be tailored to the site of perforation. If the perforation is exactly at the cardia, excision may be difficult or impossible and simple closure may provide the best result. If at all possible we attempt excision and usually do it free hand with the electrocautery. Application of clamps is difficult because of the position of the perforation. Placement of a no. 40 F Maloney dilator into the stomach will ensure that the closure retains an adequate lumen. If gastric resection is indicated, we often opt for a total gastrectomy (Chapter 25), since results are more reliable, in my opinion, than those achieved with anastomosis of the esophagus to the midstomach or distal portion of the stomach.

B. Closure may be either longitudinal along the lesser curvature, as shown here, or transverse, depending upon the site of perforation and the margins of excision. Regardless of the direction, we prefer a two-layer closure with a Connell through-and-through suture of 3-0 polyglactin (Vicryl) followed by interrupted 3-0 or 4-0 polyglactin sutures. If the lumen is narrow, it may be preferable to insert a single row of interrupted Vicryl or silk sutures.

C. If the patient is in good condition and if the site of the perforation is favorable, a distal gastric resection may be possible. The technique of resection and Billroth I anastomosis is adapted from that previously shown (see Chapter 7).

D. The extended closure of the lesser curvature may be done in two layers with a Connell suture followed by interrupted sutures or by a single row of interrupted sutures. The completed resection with the Billroth I anastomosis is shown here.

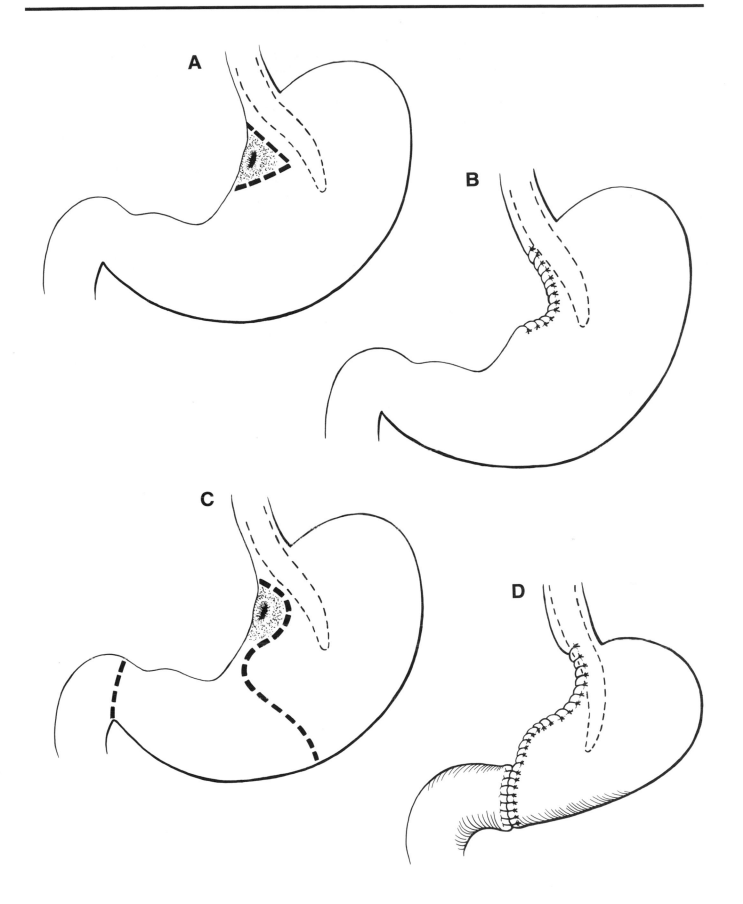

The vast majority (95%) of gastric ulcers are found in the distal stomach, so most perforated gastric ulcers are distal. These perforations may be small, pinpoint, acute prepyloric ulcers, or they may be large, thickened, and indurated, as shown in **A**. As with duodenal ulcers, most perforated gastric ulcers are anterior, since posterior ulcers tend to penetrate and fuse into the pancreas or retroperitoneum. Occasionally, however, an acute gastric ulcer will perforate posteriorly and may fill the lesser omental bursa with air. The upright radiograph may show a rectangular collection of air in the upper abdomen that on lateral view is posterior to the stomach. One problem that we face with perforated gastric ulcers that we do not face with perforations in the duodenum is the possibility of malignancy. This should be borne carefully in mind in every single patient. Each perforated gastric ulcer should be biopsied (see Chapter 7). The two options for treatment of a perforated gastric ulcer are distal gastrectomy and simple closure. The option of simple closure, of course, is available only if the gastric biopsy is negative, or if palliative treatment of a perforated gastric cancer is deemed to be the proper course because of local or systemic problems. If conditions permit, distal resection is preferable for both benign and malignant perforations. Results after resection of benign perforated gastric ulcer are far superior to those for simple closure.

FIG 20–2

A. This figure shows perforation of a large, indurated ulcer on the distal greater curvature. If frozen-section biopsy is negative, the perforation can be treated either by resection or by simple closure. Resection appears clearly to give the best long-term results and we aim for it. The duodenum is usually free and mobile and in such instances we attempt to do a 50% distal gastric resection and Billroth I anastomosis.

B. The resection and anastomosis are carried out as previously described (see Chapter 7). Occasionally, one portion of a large gastric ulcer may perforate anteriorly while another portion penetrates posteriorly into the pancreas. Mobilization of the stomach may require sharp dissection, once benignity of the ulcer has been determined. If a perforated distal gastric ulcer is shown to be malignant, we would add removal of the gastrocolic ligament and greater omentum and gastrohepatic ligament to the resection. If cure were likely, we would stay as far as possible from the tumor and obtain frozen-section biopsies of the line of resection.

C. In resections for benign ulcer we might reinforce the suture line anteriorly with a tab of omentum.

D. If decision is made not to resect the perforated ulcer, the method of closure will depend upon the size of the perforation and the induration of the surrounding gastric wall. Simple perforations may be closed and reinforced with a tab of omentum. If the perforation is large and if the walls are indurated, we usually place 2-0 silk sutures as shown here.

E. A free tab of omentum is then brought up and tied over the perforation, in a manner analogous to a Graham's closure of a perforated duodenal ulcer.

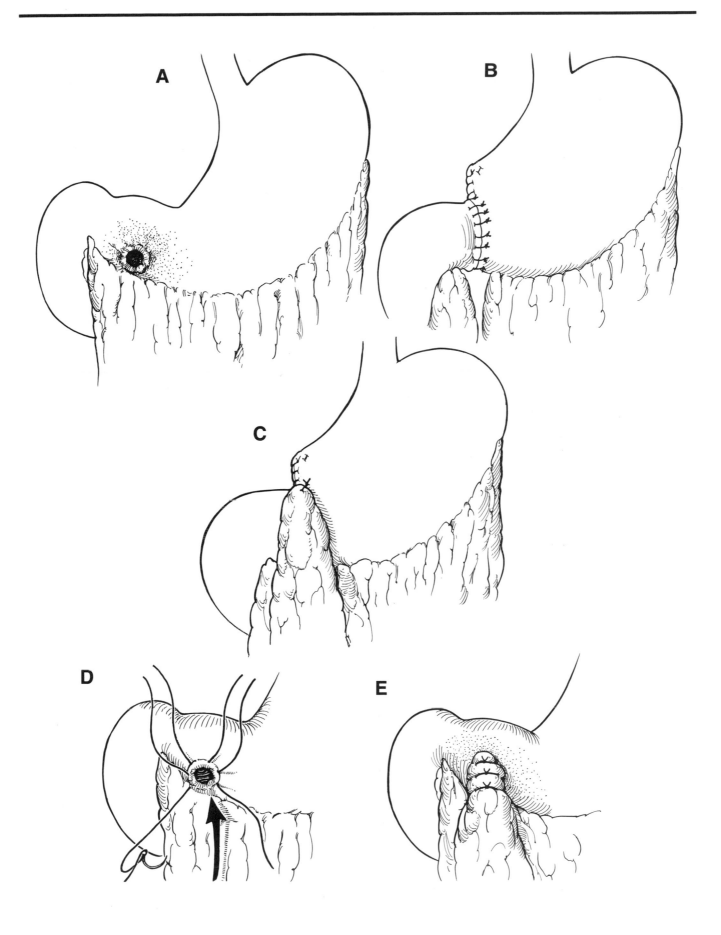

Benign Gastric Tumors

21

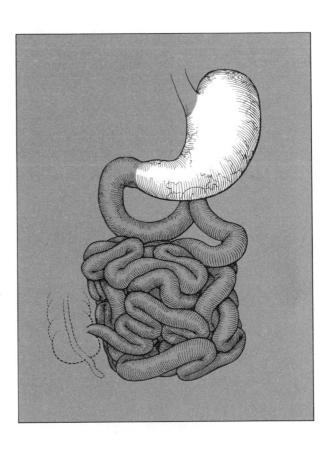

Any soft tissue tumor may occur in the stomach, but the most common are adenomas, leiomyomas, lipomas, fibromas, and angiomas. They may be sessile or polypoid; rarely they may be on a long stalk that protrudes through the pylorus and they may produce intermittent pyloric obstruction. They can almost always be diagnosed by endoscopic biopsy. If the tumor is bleeding, bleeding may be handled by electrocoagulation or heater probe through the endoscope, but if bleeding is brisk, open operation is indicated.

FIG 21-1

A. This figure shows endoscopic visualization of a leiomyoma on the posterior midgastric wall. These are typically smooth, umbilicated tumors, and they often bleed from their small volcanolike apical crater.

B. If bleeding is not brisk (some say less than 1 mL per minute) bleeding may be halted by endoscopic electrocoagulation or by use of a heater probe (tip of which is shown).

C. If bleeding is particularly brisk or if attempts at endoscopic coagulation fail, operative removal is necessary.

D. In this instance, an anterior gastrotomy should be made over the site of the posterior tumor *(dotted line)*.

E. The benign tumor is locally excised with an electrocautery.

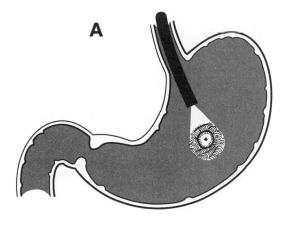

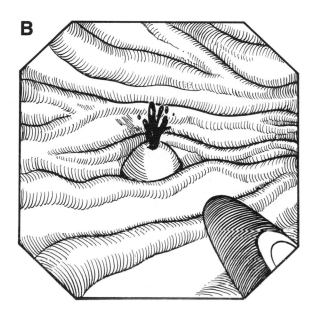

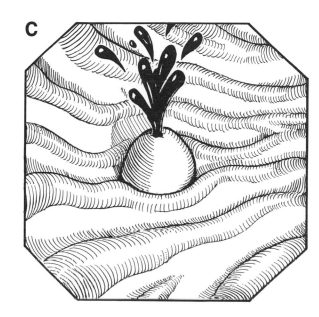

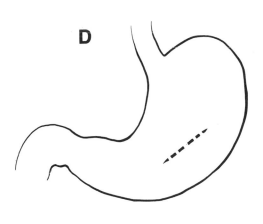

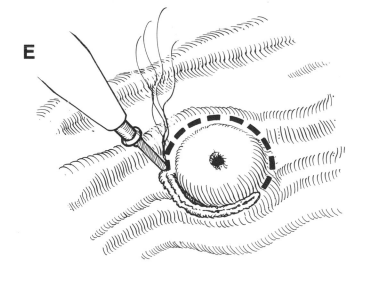

F. The arterial feeder at the base is managed by suture ligation.

G. The defect of the mucosa is closed with a simple, running suture of 4-0 polyglactin (Vicryl) and the gastrotomy closed.

H. The next two figures illustrate the case of a 49-year-old man who had undergone several episodes of massive upper gastrointestinal hemorrhage. He underwent endoscopy and a globular 2 cm tumor was found in the fundus against the posterior wall; the tumor is clearly seen in this upper gastrointestinal x-ray air-contrast study.

I. The tumor was grasped at the base, excised, and sent for frozen section and found to be a benign adenoma. The base was oversewn and the gastrotomy closed.

F

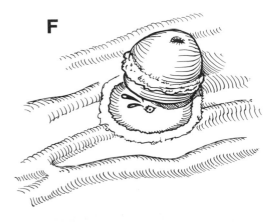

G

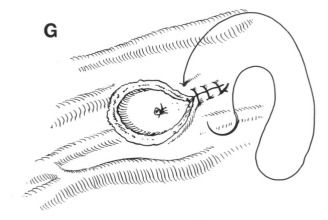

H

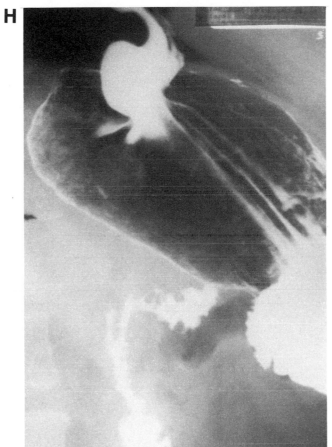

I

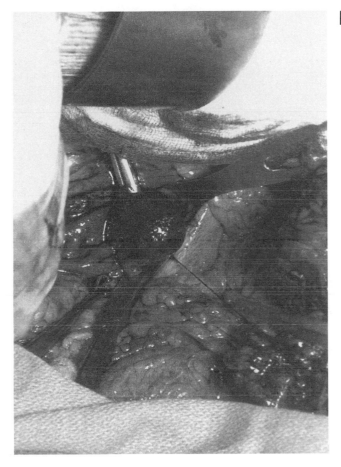

Subtotal Gastrectomy for Gastric Cancer

22

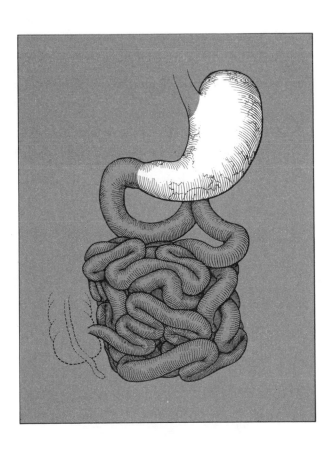

The extent of gastrectomy for gastric cancer will depend upon the site and size of the malignancy. If the entire stomach is involved, a total gastrectomy may be necessary (see Chapter 25). Any lesser involvement of the stomach usually results in subtotal gastrectomy, provided that the section of stomach to be removed may be taken out safely. If obstruction or hemorrhage is present or threatened, subtotal gastrectomy may be performed even though distant metastases are present. If a cancer exists in the distal stomach, and if the procedure is undertaken "for cure" (that is, if the surgeon believes that the tumor can be removed without gross residual), the procedure undertaken is similar to that undertaken for benign gastric ulcer, except that the lesser and greater omenta are excised, and the suture lines are usually sent to the pathology laboratory for frozen section examination to determine whether tumor is present at the line of resection. Recent experience from Japan suggests that a formal lymphadenectomy of the celiac plexus and of the lymphatics at the porta hepatis may improve cure.

FIG 22–1

A. If the tumor were prepyloric, for example, the plan would be to take the first 2 to 3 cm or so of duodenum and send the tissue at the line of resection for a frozen section biopsy. A 60% distal subtotal gastrectomy would be planned and again the line of gastric resection would be monitored by frozen section examination.

B. The greater and lesser omenta are removed by incising along the dotted lines so as to separate the greater omentum from the transverse colon inferiorly and the lesser omentum (gastrohepatic ligament) from the liver. The greater omentum is almost always best removed from left to right, going along the relatively avascular plane of attachment to the transverse colon. Great care should be taken here to avoid injury to the middle colic artery and vein. We try carefully to avoid hematomas, which may obscure the position of the vessels, although the pulsating artery is usually easily palpated from the inferior aspect of the transverse mesocolon. In excising the gastrohepatic and hepatoduodenal ligaments (which together form the lesser omentum), dissection should again be carried out from left to right—in this instance, just below the attachment to the liver. At the extreme right, care is needed to avoid biliary injury.

C. Once the attachment of the greater omentum to the colon has been severed, the omentum and gastrocolic ligament are lifted anteriorly, taking care again to avoid injury to the middle colic vessels. Occasionally, the gastrocolic ligament and transverse mesocolon will be fused and require separation by sharp dissection. The greater and lesser omenta are left attached to the gastric specimen. If a subtotal gastrectomy is planned, the greater and lesser omenta are separated from the proximal stomach that will remain.

D. A Billroth II anastomosis is almost always preferable in patients with distal gastric cancer so that a local recurrence will not cause gut obstruction. The gastrojejunostomy should be placed on the greater curvature proximal to the closure of the stomach so as to avoid any potential closure of the anastomosis by a recurrence of the tumor.

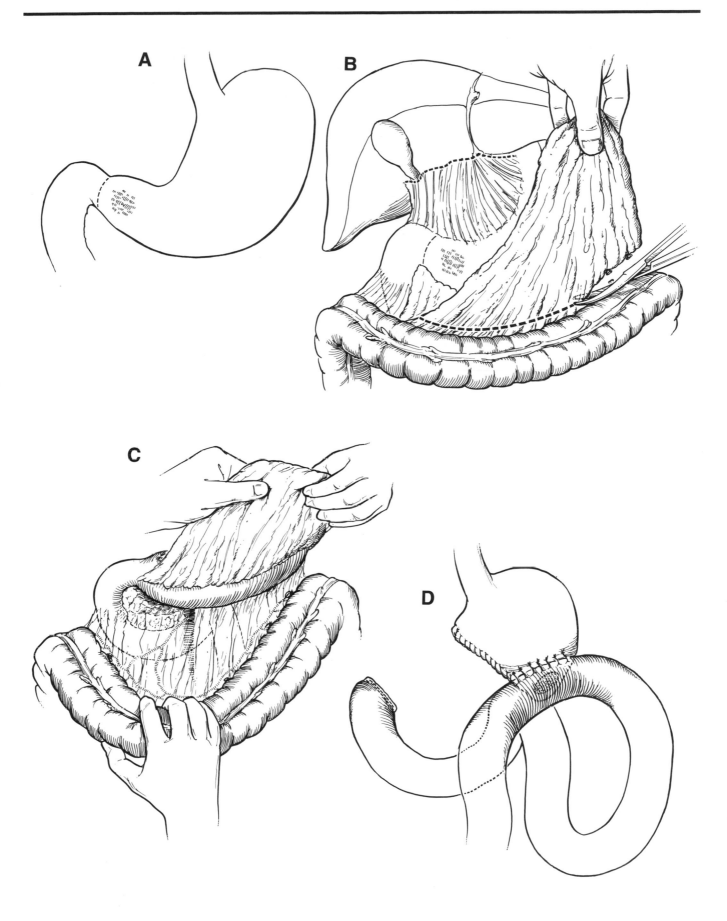

Palliative Bypass for Gastric Cancer

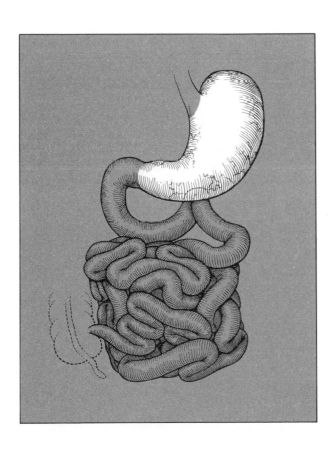

FIG 23–1

By the time patients with gastric cancer seek medical help they often have a far-advanced tumor, and symptoms of obstruction are often the problem that brings the patient to see the physician. Barium x-ray and endoscopic examination will allow an evaluation of whether or not obstruction exists. The decision as to whether or not a tumor can be resected is usually made at operation. Excision of the tumor is clearly preferable even if there is no chance of its eradication, since its removal will diminish the chances of later hemorrhage, perforation, or reobstruction.

Local spread of the tumor to retroperitoneal structures (e.g., common bile duct, portal vein, and pancreas), however, has often advanced to the point that any attempt at excision would be dangerous. This problem is usually best solved by a simple gastrojejunostomy with an anastomosis proximal to the tumor. If, however, the lesion has been bleeding, we often open the stomach, attempt to ligate the area of bleeding, and may even attempt to partially devascularize the stomach by ligating the appropriate arteries (for example, with bleeding from a distal nonresectable cancer, we might ligate the right and left gastric and the right and left gastroepiploic arteries). Unfortunately, these maneuvers often fail; if bleeding is persistent, a palliative resection (if at all feasible) may be necessary. The loop of jejunum is brought up and anastomosed to the stomach. The anastomosis should be sufficiently distant from the tumor so as to avoid future obstruction and sufficiently distal in location on the stomach itself so as to provide drainage that is as complete as possible. Choice of anterior or posterior gastroenterostomy may depend entirely upon the preference of the surgeon unless there is a greater anterior or posterior extent of the tumor, in which case the anastomosis should properly be placed on the opposite side.

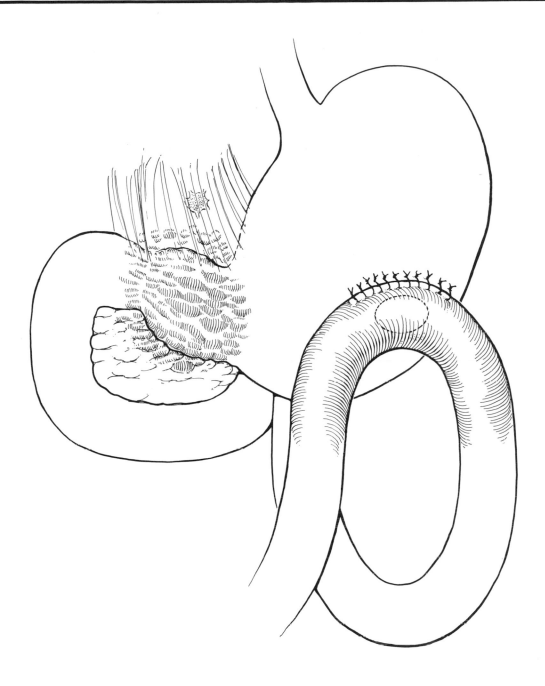

Gastric Barosurgery
(Bypass and Gastroplasty)

24

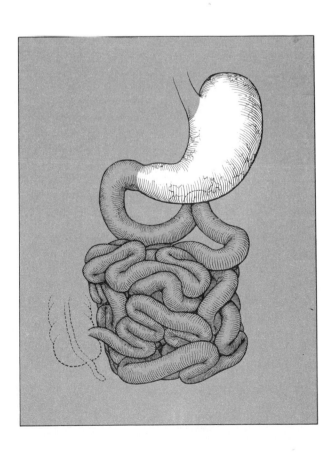

Surgeons are endlessly inventive. When a demand rose to assist morbidly obese people to lose weight, the procedure of jejunoileal bypass was devised and was popular for several years. Severe metabolic sequelae and several deaths quelled enthusiasm. Mason at Iowa introduced procedures to bypass all but a small gastric pouch, thereby reducing the amount anyone could eat at one time. Several procedures for gastric barosurgery have evolved. I will describe here gastric bypass and vertical banded gastroplasty. I no longer do barosurgery, but the procedures are popular and often successful. Anyone who has operated upon morbidly obese persons knows that the major problem faced during such operation is exposure. Big incisions, deep retractors, and experienced and talented assistants are necessary. The distal esophagus and proximal stomach should be mobilized. The uppermost vasa brevia may be divided, depending upon how much exposure of the upper greater curvature of the stomach is required.

FIG 24–1

A.   In performing a gastric bypass, the essential maneuver is to construct a proximal gastric pouch that will contain between 30 and 60 mL. The distal esophagus and proximal stomach are completely mobilized. The TA-90 stapler should be placed by first extending the anvil. Pulling the anvil through posterior to the stomach can be facilitated by inserting the end of the anvil into a large mushroom catheter previously placed behind the stomach. When positioning the ends of the stapler on the lesser curvature, care should be taken to protect the vagus nerves by pulling them to the right, away from the jaws of the stapler. The stapling device is approximated and closed, but not fired. An Ewald tube is placed into the small proximal pouch and a Penrose drain is placed around the distal esophagus and clamped tightly, so as to occlude the esophagus around the Ewald tube. By first measuring the volume of dead space in the Ewald tube itself, placement of fluid through the tube into the gastric pouch will allow for measurement of the pouch volume. If volume is incorrect, the stapler can be moved. Once the desired volume (30 to 60 mL) is achieved, the pouch is emptied, the Penrose drain around the esophagus is removed, and the stapler is fired. Some surgeons like to place another row of staples side-by-side, so as to minimize the risk of leakage.

B.   The proximal jejunum is mobilized and brought anterior to the colon. A posterior row of interrupted 4-0 polyglactin Vicryl sutures is placed and the adjacent walls of the stomach and jejunum are opened by electrocautery dissection. Hemostasis is secured and a through-and-through suture is effected by means of two swaged 3-0 polyglactin sutures placed in a running locking fashion posteriorly and then brought around anteriorly in a Connell suture. The aperture should be small, just about 1 cm. The anastomosis is completed with an anterior row of polyglactin sutures. Some surgeons prefer to use a Roux-en-Y limb for the anastomosis between the stomach and jejunum. This has the potential hazard of subjecting the unbuffered jejunal mucosa to the direct effect of gastric acid. Although early results with gastric bypass are usually good, the pouch often expands and the patient gains weight later. Another common problem is spontaneous opening of the staple line, which has led some surgeons, as noted above, to use four rows of staples. Because of the problems with gastric bypass, another method for diminishing the size of the gastric reservoir, the vertical banded gastroplasty, was developed.

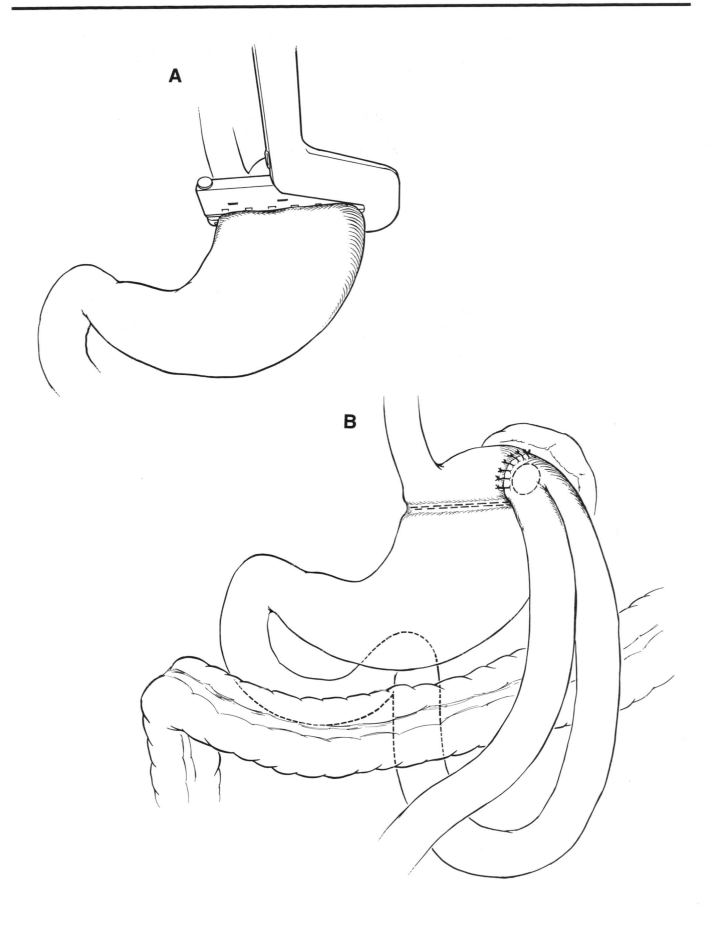

C. Performance of the vertical banded gastroplasty requires mobilization of the proximal stomach and intra-abdominal esophagus, as described above. A large intraluminal tube is placed along the lesser curvature, so as to preserve the lumen. Some use a no. 32 F Maloney dilator, others use a no. 32 F Ewald tube, which is later used for calibration of the size of the pouch (the ideal pouch size is 30 to 50 mL). Probably the best way to get the post of the EEA stapling device through both walls of the stomach is to take a metal trocar and fit the blunt end to a soft rubber tube, the diameter of which will fit the post of the EEA stapling device snugly. The trocar is then passed through both walls of the stomach with the Maloney dilator in place. The post of the extended EEA stapler is then fitted into the end of the rubber tubing protruding through the anterior gastric wall and the post pulled through both front and back walls of the stomach. Once the post is through the posterior wall, the tubing is removed and the anvil inserted onto the post, as shown. The anvil and stapling device are then approximated, the stapler fired, the anvil is then distracted and removed. The stomach now has a circular aperture with two circumferential rows of staples. The stapling device should be disassembled and two intact rings of gastric wall retrieved.

D. This figure shows that the inferior aspect of the tunnel along the lesser curvature of the stomach has been occluded by means of tension on a through-and-through Penrose drain placed through the aperture created by the EEA stapling device. The drain is tightened and held in place with a clamp. The Ewald tube is brought just through the cardia and a Penrose drain tightened about it. In order to place the TA-90 stapling device for the vertical band of staples, a no. 30 chest tube is then placed behind the stomach through the EEA aperture and passed upwards towards the angle of His, and brought around behind the stomach. The tip of the anvil of the TA-90 stapling device is then placed in the open end of the chest tube and gently manipulated behind the stomach. When the hub of the TA-90 stapler is seated within the gastric window, the stapling device is then closed so as to allow measurement of the size of the pouch. When an appropriate size (30 to 50 mL) has been achieved, the stapler is fired, opened, and removed. Another TA-90 stapling device is then placed in the same position, but just to the left, and fired again so as to achieve four parallel staple lines.

E. This figure shows the lesser curvature tunnel, with the four lines of staples. In order to prevent the lower aperture of the pouch from stretching, a narrow (1.5 cm) strip of Marlex mesh is passed through it and the no. 32 F Maloney dilator then passed through the tunnel.

F. The mesh is then sewn tightly together so as to create approximately a 5 cm circumferential outer band.

G. After the vertical banded gastroplasty is finished, some surgeons place a tab of omentum over the gastric aperture, some do not.

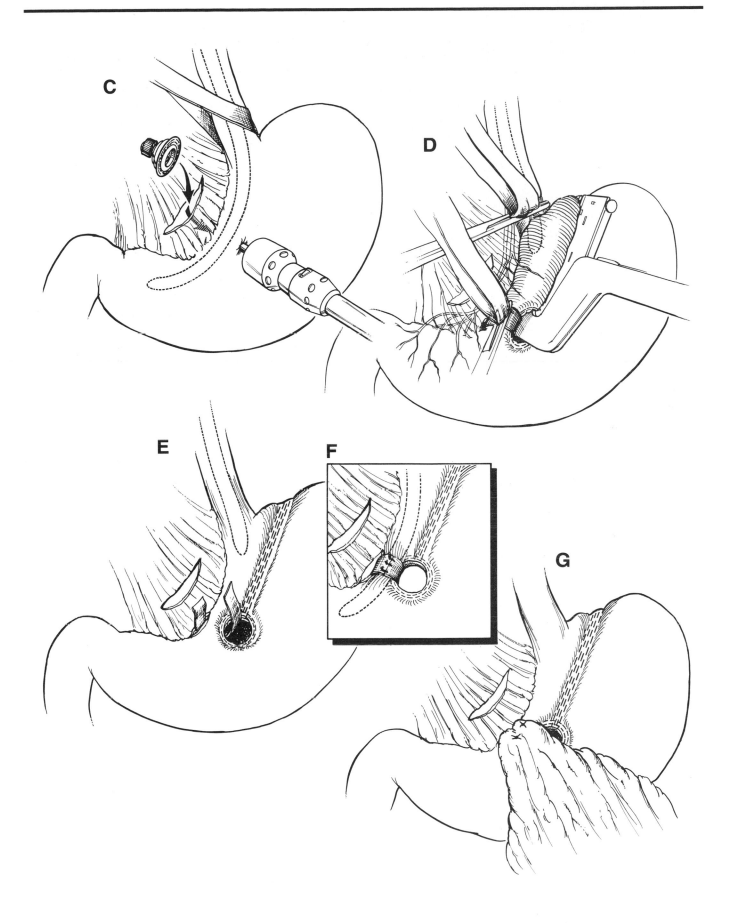

Total Gastrectomy

25

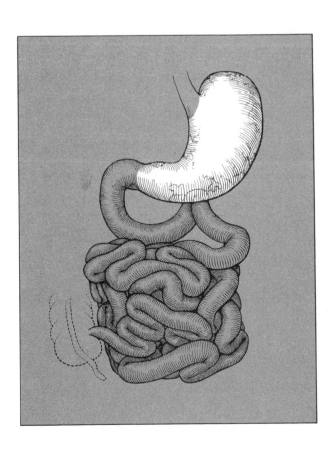

Total gastrectomy may be performed for benign or malignant lesions. In terms of peptic ulcer disease, total gastrectomy is the ultimate operation, since it totally defuses the problem of peptic ulcer and is curative for the hypersecretory aspects of the Zollinger-Ellison syndrome. We and others (some of whom refer to the procedure euphemistically as completion gastrectomy) have used it infrequently in order to manage patients with virulent, nongastrinoma, recurrent peptic ulcer disease that has persisted despite multiple previous operations of resection and vagotomy. In patients with diffuse hemorrhagic gastritis that has resisted all local and pharmacologic treatment, total gastrectomy provides the one sure method for halting bleeding. We may, rarely, perform total gastrectomy for trauma or for gastric necrosis after toxic ingestion (of large amounts of strong acid, for example). Most experience with total gastrectomy is in patients with malignant disease, where it is of great use in patients with massive gastric lymphoma, with widespread superficial spreading gastric carcinoma, and with tumors of the body of the stomach that progress proximally and distally. Cure rates in operating upon huge tumors are not great, but in patients in whom there has been submucosal spread of relatively small tumors, total gastrectomy provides the best chance for surgical cure. Total gastrectomy for malignancies combines resection of the entire stomach along with removal of the gastrohepatic ligament and the gastrocolic ligament. The spleen is often taken when tumors involve the gastric fundus.

Total gastrectomy is often performed in patients who have not had previous gastric operations, but it is often performed on patients who have had multiple previous gastric procedures. The operation illustrated here is a first-time resection. The procedure shown initially is for removal of benign lesions, after which the excision of the gastrohepatic and gastrocolic ligaments for cancer is illustrated. We have routinely used a Roux-en-Y esophagojejunostomy for reconstruction after total gastrectomy. Another alternative is the interposition of a free jejunal segment as an end-to-end conduit between the esophagus and duodenum. We have been so pleased with our long-term results with the Roux-en-Y that we have no experience with the interposition method; the good results recently reported from Northern Germany with interposition suggest that it may be as good as or even superior to the Roux-en-Y. Other considerations in patients with Zollinger-Ellison syndrome, such as diagnosis, consideration of therapeutic alternatives, technique and search for gastrinomas, and the management of a solitary gastrinoma, for example, extend beyond the scope of this work. I would like to stress that regardless of how the hypersecretory aspects of the gastrinoma syndrome are managed, all patients have tumors that are potentially malignant and therefore all patients should be operated upon unless there is some contraindication, such as widespread metastasis and imminent death. As Zollinger has repeatedly pointed out, we operate on any other endocrine tumor of the pancreas. The cure rates for gastrinoma are well within those for other intra-abdominal malignancies that we routinely operate upon. Stabile and Passaro and their colleagues have pointed out that the vast majority of gastrinomas are found within a triangle bounded superiorly by the cystic duct, medially by the neck of the pancreas, and inferiorly by the junction of the second and third part of the duodenum. This area should be carefully searched in all patients with gastrinomas. We and others have found that any gastrinoma that is extrapancreatic and extraintestinal is apt to be solitary, and its removable is apt to produce cure. Total gastrectomy has fallen out of favor with most physicians who treat patients with the Zollinger-Ellison tumor because of the efficacy of the H_2-receptor antagonists, and especially of the proton-pump blocker, omeprazole. The drugs are extraordinary effective and very few patients are, in fact, resistant to omeprazole therapy. Our problem in managing these patients has been in their compliance (that is, in their failure to adhere to long-term programs of medication), and, since the symptoms are often cyclic, many patients will stop taking their medications at a time when the disease is in spontaneous remission. Since nothing happens, they continue to abstain from drug therapy. The disease may then recur with sudden ferocity, causing bleeding or proliferation or massive hypersecretion. The last 18 patients we have operated on had stopped taking their medications. We performed total gastrectomy in the initial patients we treated for the Zollinger-Ellison syndrome and we are satisfied with its results. We have done 36 total gastrectomies on patients with the Zollinger-Ellison syndrome without mortality, and they have a surprisingly good nutritional response to total gastrectomy. In sum, we have been pleased with the results of the procedure, and if our patients remember to take their vitamin B$_{12}$ injections, we have few sequelae. Dumping is unusually infrequent (only three of our patients have been greatly troubled and all openly responded to inclusion of dietary resin). Weight loss of more than 20% is rare, unless the patient should develop widespread metastatic disease. We first illustrate total gastrectomy for benign (noncancerous) diseases, and then total gastrectomy for malignancy.

Total Gastrectomy for Benign Disease

FIG 25–1

A. This figure illustrates mobilization of the stomach by serial division of the vessels in the gastrocolic ligament and in the gastrohepatic ligament so as to entirely free up the greater and lesser curvatures. The short gastric vessels connecting the stomach to the spleen have been divided and the spleen preserved. The stomach should be lifted anteriorly so as to free it from any posterior connections to the pancreas or retroperitoneum.

B. The duodenum is divided just distal to the pylorus. The division can be made between Kocher clamps as shown here, to be followed with a suture closure of the duodenal stump (see Chapter 9). If, however, the duodenum is free of any disease (especially severe fibrosis) that might make a staple closure insecure, we are more apt to use the staple closure of the duodenum (see Chapter 9). The proximal line of division should be in the distal intra-abdominal esophagus. When removing the stomach for peptic ulcer disease (the Zollinger-Ellison syndrome or recurrent marginal ulceration), care should be taken to remove all fundic mucosa. In such instances, we routinely get a frozen section biopsy of the end of the esophagus, just to be sure that there are no acid-secreting glands left.

C. After the gastric specimen is removed and the duodenal stump closed, we direct attention to the intra-abdominal esophagus. We put in a free-hand through-and-through running pursestring stitch, using a swaged heavy prolene suture. We do not use the pursestring suture clamp device, since it often fails. We then estimate the size of the distal esophagus using sizing gauges, as shown here. These sizers must be used with care; excess force will split the esophagus. The end-to-end anastomotic stapling device usually comes in three sizes, and we can usually get the medium sizer into the lower esophagus. In patients with the Zollinger-Ellison syndrome, however, we almost never can get anything larger than the small. Because of this, we have had three or four patients who have had some dysphagia after esophagojejunostomy. Fortunately, this responds well to esophageal dilatation by bougienage, and we have never had to perform dilatation on anyone more than twice.

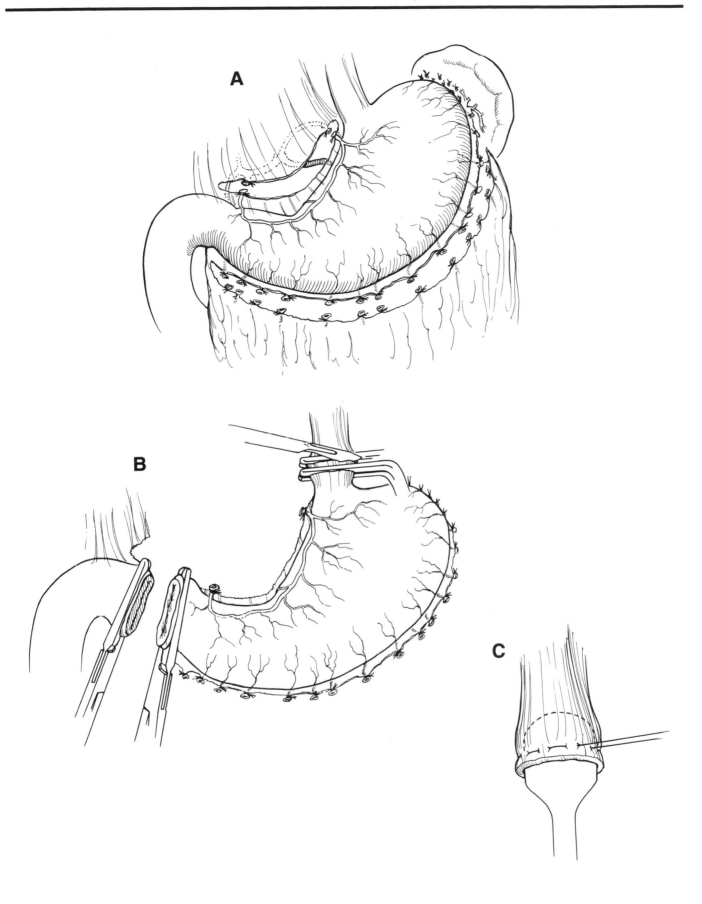

A

B

C

D. The next step is to mobilize and divide the proximal jejunum. We select a segment of jejunum 12 to 15 cm distal to the ligament of Treitz and, after inspection of the vascular arcade so as to be certain that we can easily mobilize the distal limb up to the esophagus, we divide the jejunum (shown here between Kocher clamps). We now usually do this division with the GIA stapling device (see Fig. **42–4, O,** p. 000). The proximal end of the jejunum, marked *b,* is left in situ and the distal end, marked *a,* is brought up through a rent in the transverse mesocolon (made with care so as to avoid injury to the middle colic vessels), along a path shown by the *arrows,* so as to approximate the esophagus.

E. Stay sutures are placed on the free end of the jejunum *(a),* and the EEA stapling device (without the anvil) is placed into the lumen of the free end of the jejunum. If the jejunum has been divided with the GIA stapler, the jejunum is opened adjacent to the line of staples, and the EEA device (without anvil) is inserted. A point is selected about 4 to 5 cm from the free margin and the extended post of the EEA device is brought through the wall of the jejunum. In doing this, we usually press the post against the wall and make a small opening with the electrocautery and push the post on through. This obviates the need for a jejunal pursestring suture.

F. The anvil is then screwed onto the extended post and inserted into the distal esophagus.

G. This figure shows in cross section the beginning approximation of the esophagus (with the pursestring tied and knotted) and the jejunum. Further approximation brings the anvil down onto the EEA stapler which is then fired. Firing of the stapler simultaneously places a circular double ring of staples and extends a circular knife that excises the rings of the jejunum and esophagus inside the circle of staples. The large wing nut on the end of the EEA stapling device is then opened so as to disapproximate the anvil and stapler and the anvil is gently maneuvered out through the new anastomosis between the esophagus and jejunum.

H. The stapler is then disassembled so as to allow inspection of the rings (doughnuts) of esophageal and jejunal walls. Both rings must be intact or the anastomosis must be done again.

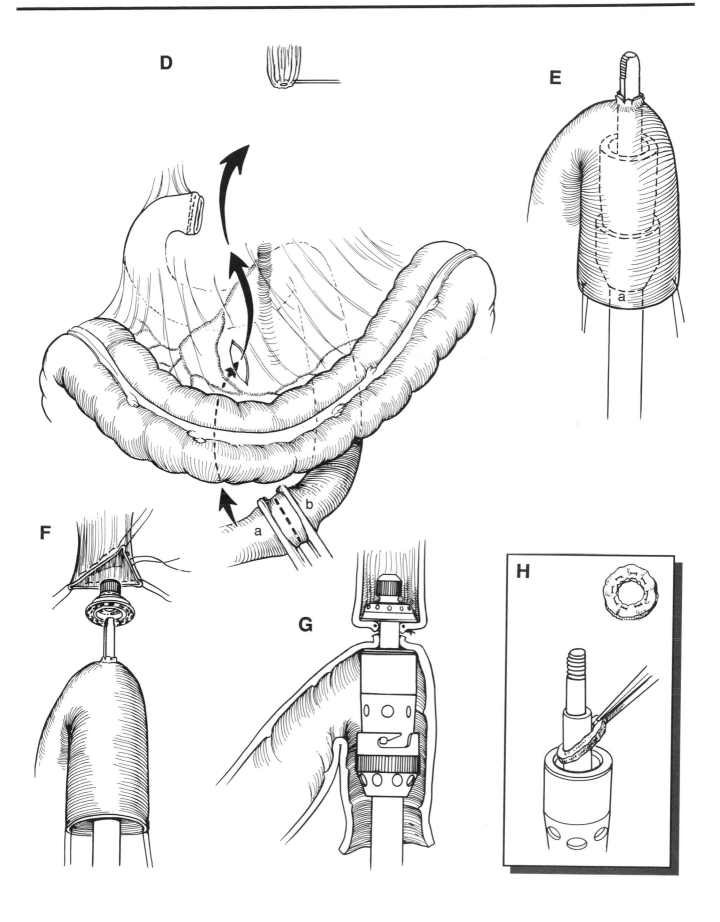

D

E

F

G

H

Total Gastrectomy

I.   This shows excision of the redundant segment of jejunum beyond the esophagojejunostomy. The TA-55 stapling device is placed and the staples fired, and the redundant segment of jejunum is removed. This converts the anastomosis functionally into an end-to-end esophagojejunostomy (see **L**).

J.   The continuity of the bowel is then restored with a jejunojejunostomy to complete the Roux-en-Y. We approximate the two limbs of jejunum with a suture, make openings in each limb with an electrocautery, and insert the two limbs of the GIA stapling device. After making sure that the tips are free, the device is fired and removed. This creates a stapled opening between the two limbs of the jejunum.

K.   The openings made in the two limbs are then closed transversely with a TA-55 stapling device, holding the free margins together with a row of Babcock clamps. After the stapler is fired, protruding tissue in the Babcock clamp is excised with a Mayo scissors.

L.   This figure shows a completed operation. We show in this instance a stapled duodenal stump and a stapled jejunojejunostomy. The length of jejunum between the esophagojejunostomy and the jejunojejunostomy should be 40 to 50 cm. We have had reflux of bile into the esophagus in some patients with a 40 cm loop, and in those patients we have revised the loop to 60 cm. We have lately constructed 50 cm limbs so as to diminish the risk of bile reflux esophagitis.

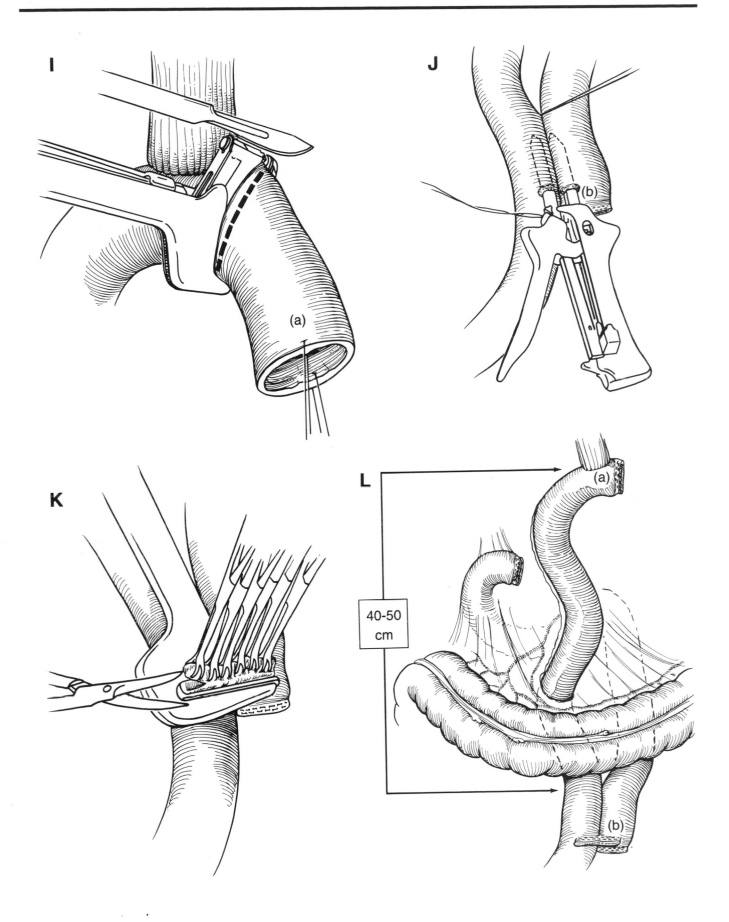

Total Gastrectomy for Malignancy

When performing a total gastrectomy for cancer, it is necessary to mobilize all potential lymph node–bearing tissue prior to dissecting the stomach itself for total gastrectomy. The technique is otherwise similar to that of total gastrectomy for benign disease. Similar resection of the gastrocolic and gastrohepatic ligaments should, of course, accompany subtotal gastrectomy for cancer.

FIG 25–2

A. Dissection is best accomplished by total excision of the gastrocolic ligament and the gastrohepatic ligament. Japanese surgeons point out the value of a formal celiac and portal lymphadenectomy, but most American surgeons simply remove both omenta. The gastrocolic ligament is best removed by grasping the left margin and dividing its relatively avascular attachments to the transverse colon. The surgeon should be on guard against possible fusion of the gastrocolic ligament and the transverse mesocolon, in which case the vessels to the transverse colon might be accidentally injured. Injury to colonic vessels is best avoided by first dividing the avascular attachments and then placing traction on the transverse colon and ligating any small vessels in the gastrocolic ligament attached to the transverse colon. The right side is often more vascular and requires more dissection to separate the gastrocolic ligament from the transverse mesocolon. Injury to colonic vessels may occur during this resection when the surgeon fails to anticipate fusion. The gastrohepatic ligament is best divided at its attachments to the liver, taking care to avoid injury to the portal structures and gallbladder. The left gastric artery is divided near to its origin from the celiac.

B. After the gastrocolic ligament has been divided from its attachment to the transverse colon, the entire greater omentum can then be lifted along with the stomach to visualize the lesser omental bursa. The retrogastric area should be carefully inspected for possible involvement with tumor. If the spleen appears to be adjacent to or involved in tumor, the splenic artery and vein can be divided at some distance from the splenic hilum and the spleen can be removed with the stomach. Similarly, possible invasion of the tail of pancreas can be managed by performing a distal pancreatic resection and delivering the tail of the pancreas and spleen along with the stomach.

C. This shows the completed operation with a stapled duodenal stump and esophagojejunostomy, and a sutured jejunojejunostomy. The 40 to 50 cm length of the Roux-en-Y limb is necessary to prevent bile reflux into the esophagus. Another option is to perform a stapled jejunojejunostomy as illustrated under total gastrectomy for benign disease (see **Fig 25–1,** J–L; p. 161).

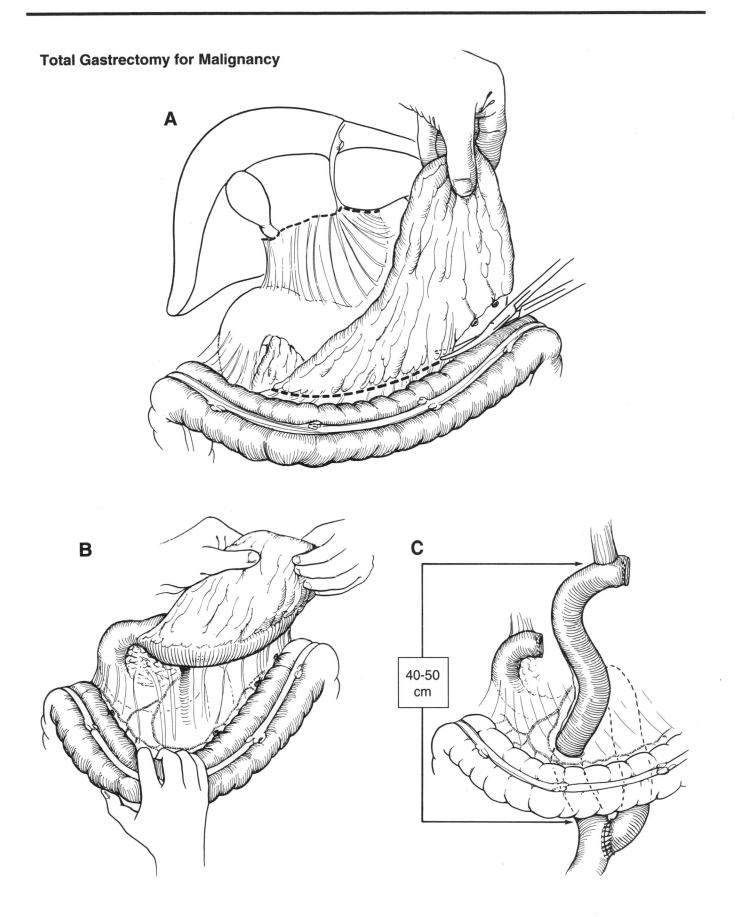

Modified EEA Stapling Device

FIG 25–3

A. New instruments appear all the time and a recent modification of the EEA stapler may facilitate the performance of the esophagojejunostomy. The principles are the same, but the interlocking process between anvil and stapler may be more easily achieved. In this illustration, the disposable plastic trocar attached to the anvil protrudes through the jejunal wall. After protrusion, the post of the anvil is extended and the trocar discarded.

B. A new piece (marked by the star) is an interlocking post which fits upward into the new capped anvil, and which protrudes downward to fit, male into female as it were, into the protruding post of the stapler.

C. This figure shows a cross section of the esophagojejunostomy that is about to be created. The interlocking post has been reeled into the stapler and the stapler and anvil (with the end of the esophagus cinched up below it by means of the pursestring suture) are approximated. The stapler is fired, the circular knife cuts out the rings of jejunum and esophagus, and the staples and anvil are distracted and gently removed. The redundant jejunum is excised as in **Fig 25–1, I** (p. 161), converting the anastomosis functionally to end-to-end. The jejunojunostomy completes the Roux-en-Y.

D. After removing the EEA stapler, the surgeon must check the integrity of the esophageal and jejunal "doughnuts."

Modified EEA Stapling Device

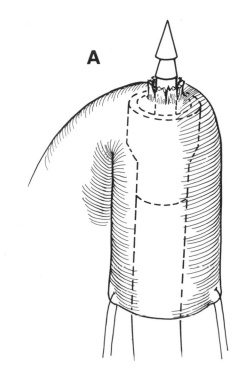

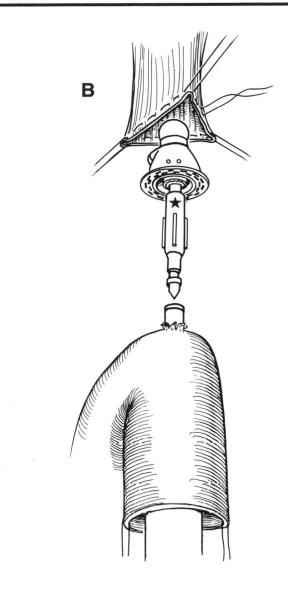

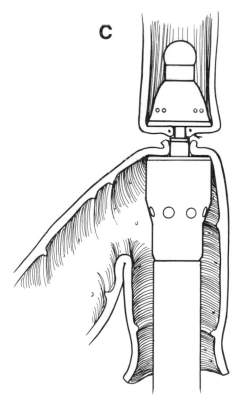

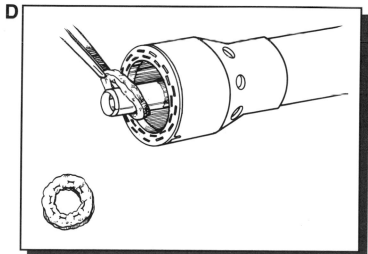

Complications
of Gastric Operations

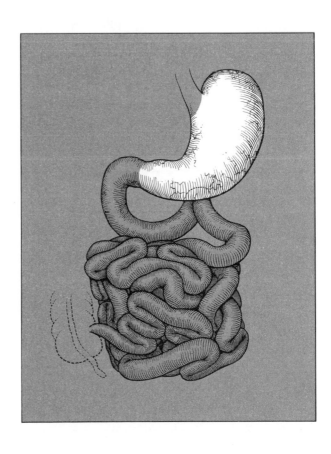

26

Early Complications: Postoperative Hemorrhage Managed by Endoscopy

The vast majority of early postgastrectomy hemorrhage is due to bleeding from suture lines. Every surgeon should heed this knowledge, and should carefully inspect suture lines before closing the lumen. Persistent bleeding from the nasogastric tube after operation should alert the surgeon to the possibility of suture line hemorrhage. Although we often allow duodenal ulcer craters to remain in situ after gastrectomy (even when the indication for operation has been hemorrhage), persistent or recurrent hemorrhage from the ulcer is not the usual cause of postoperative bleeding, although it must be considered. Careful application of the U-stitch technique (see Chapter 17) has greatly decreased the incidence of recurrent ulcer bleeding after operation. Many, perhaps most, episodes of postoperative suture line bleeding can be managed endoscopically. The therapeutic choices are local injection of a vasoconstrictor (epinephrine, 1:1,000), laser photocoagulation or local coagulation by means of a heater probe. My colleague, William H. Nealon, M.D., our Chief of Endoscopy, prefers local injection of epinephrine.

FIG 26—1

A. After diagnosis of bleeding from the suture line by endoscopy, attempts are made to evacuate any blood that has collected around the bleeding point. This is usually accomplished by vigorous irrigation. The sclerotherapy needle shown in this illustration has emerged through the port of the endoscope and has been advanced so as to insert the needle adjacent to the point of bleeding.

B. Multiple injections of small volumes of vasoconstrictor at the points indicated usually are effective in stanching the hemorrhage. Injection of excess vasoconstrictor may cause an ulceration, whereas an insufficient dose may allow bleeding to continue. Injections should be in 0.1 mL increments, with a maximal dose of 1.0 mL (success is usually achieved with less).

C. Use of the heater probe may be impossible if bleeding is excessive. If it is possible to get the tip of the probe adjacent to the point of bleeding, application of heat will often be effective in halting the bleeding. High-flow irrigation is incorporated into one of the channels of the heater probe catheter, which greatly facilitates visualization.

D. Both the argon and the Nd-YAG laser may be used for treatment of postoperative bleeding. In practice, however, the method has few advantages and is cumbersome and hazardous. If the laser is used, the laser energy should not be focused on the point of bleeding. Rather, multiple points around the bleeding site should be treated by photocoagulation.

E. This figure is an enlargement of the different tips (needle, laser, and heater probe units) that go through the ports of the endoscope.

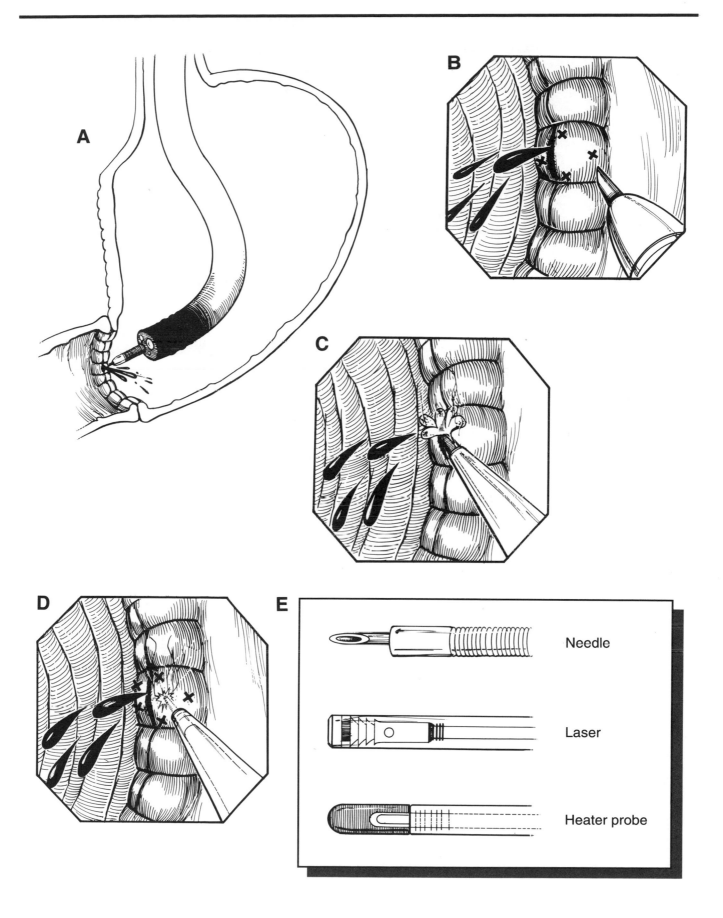

Early Complications: Postoperative Hemorrhage Managed by Operation

Most postoperative bleeding can be managed endoscopically (see **Fig. 26–1**). Should endoscopic maneuvers prove inadequate, it may be necessary to operate on the patient. The surgeon should know the site of bleeding from endoscopic examination.

FIG 26–2

A. In the event that bleeding follows a subtotal gastrectomy and gastroduodenostomy, and in the event that, say, the bleeding was found by endoscopy to come from the posterior aspect of the anastomotic suture line, a gastrotomy would be made along the *dotted line*.

B. Traction on the distal end of the incision with a vein retractor reveals the site of hemorrhage, which is treated by insertion of local sutures. When hemostasis has been well secured, the gastrotomy wound is closed. We often place a pad of omentum over the closure to prevent a leak.

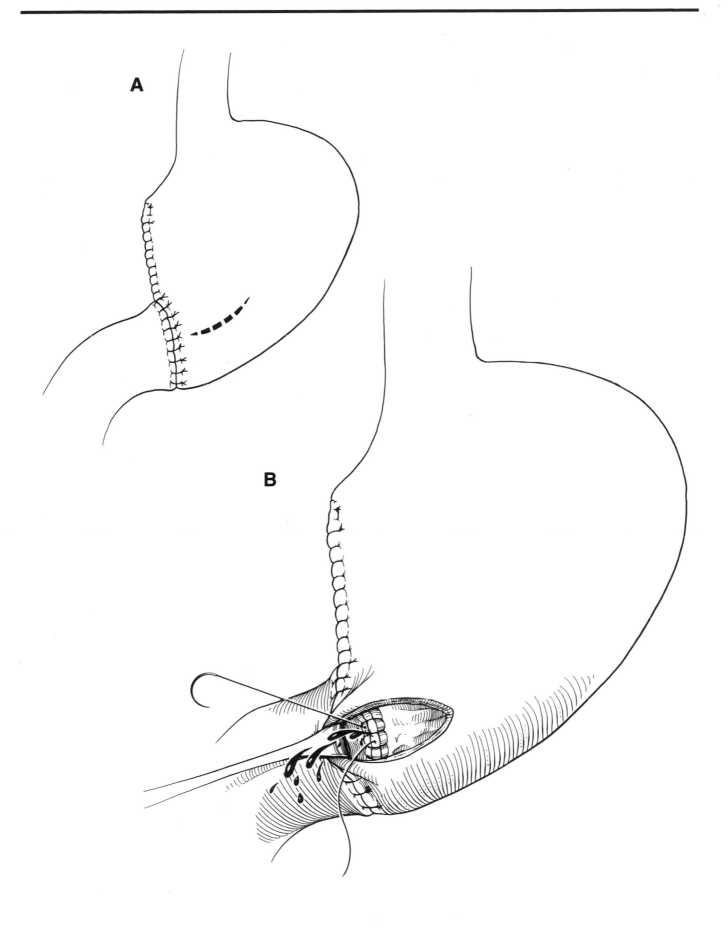

Early Complications: Leaking Anastomosis

Among the most dreaded complications of gastric resection are leaking anastomoses, usually either a leaking gastroduodenostomy (from a Billroth I procedure) or a leaking duodenal stump (Billroth II). The leak occurs because the duodenum is inflamed or fibrotic or both, and is often unsuited for anastomosis or closure. A duodenum that is badly scarred or inflamed sends a clear danger signal and the surgeon is well advised to avoid opening it; avoidance can be achieved by performing either a vagotomy and gastroenterostomy or a selective proximal vagotomy. If the indication for operation is hemorrhage, the duodenum *must* be opened; we usually prefer pyloroplasty with suture ligation of the bleeding vessel and truncal vagotomy. Pyloroplasty closures of badly scarred duodenal bulbs may leak. (An insecure pyloroplasty closure may be an indication for placing a tab of omentum over the pyloroplasty.) Leaks from gastrojejunal anastomoses are rare, since both gastric and jejunal tissues are normal (unscarred). If a gastrojejunostomy should leak, early repair can be accomplished by local suture plus an omental tab buttress. If the diagnosis is made late and tissues are inflamed and edematous, repair is hazardous and the treatment choice is between attempts at repair (possibly with excision of old anastomosis and performing a new one) or extensive local suction drainage with long-term nasogastric suction and enteral feeding (tube into midjejunum) or parenteral nutrition. The event that signals a leaking gastroduodenostomy or a leaking duodenal stump is a sudden change in the patient's clinical status, with upper abdominal pain, tenderness, and muscle guarding. Suspicions may be confirmed radiographically by gastrograffin swallow or by endoscopy, but the abrupt alteration of the patient's course alone often gives a clear clue. Treatment requires reoperation.

FIG 26–3

A. A leaking gastroduodenostomy causes edema and inflammation of the distal stomach and proximal duodenum, often with great swelling. The cause of the leak is usually local ischemia. A disrupted suture may be seen. Closure is difficult because of the extent of inflammation. The problem is probably best handled by application of a buttress, either a serosal patch or omentum.

B. This figure shows closure of the leak with an omental patch and proximate placement of a Jackson-Pratt drain.

C. Leakage of the duodenal stump was formerly the bête noire of the gastric surgeon. The complication often persists as a duodenal fistula and has a high risk of mortality. The local duodenal tissue is often so edematous and inflamed as to discourage any attempt at local suture.

D. Best results are probably secured by an omental or serosal patch and placement of a Jackson-Pratt drain immediately adjacent to the closure so as to provide for a controlled fistula should the leak recur. If the leak does persist, the drainage catheter should be left in for an extended period. A sealed drainage tract will result, which will usually close spontaneously.

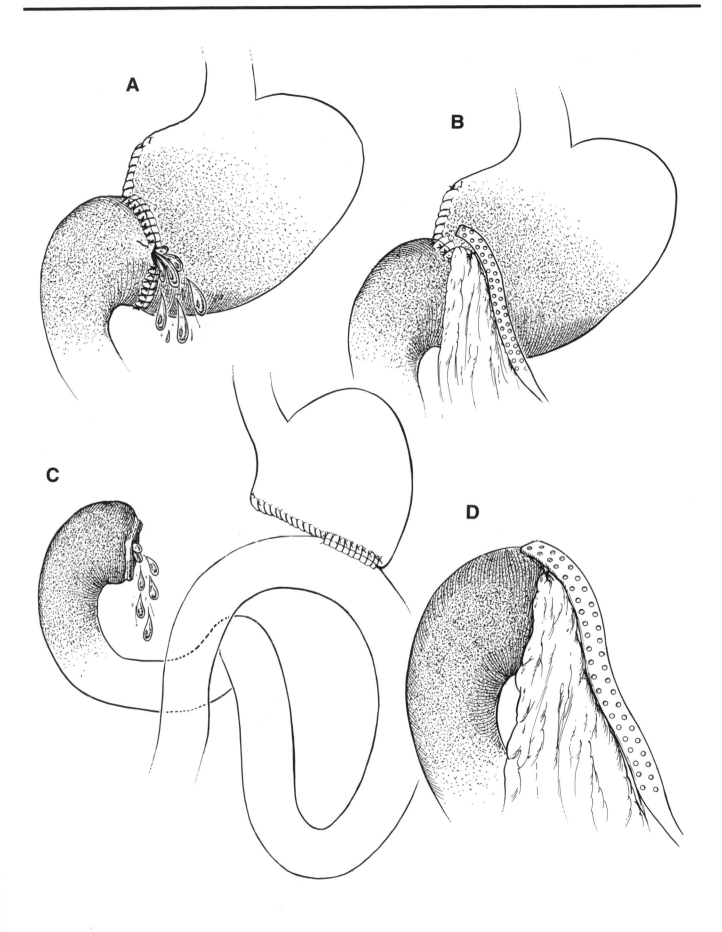

Late Complications: Recurrent Peptic Ulcer

The rate of ulcer recurrence after operation for peptic ulcer varies according to the original site of ulcer and according to the operation performed. Duodenal ulcer recurs more often than does gastric ulcer, and recurrent duodenal ulcers are more common after the conservative operations of vagotomy and drainage or selective proximal vagotomy. Conservative operations have a lower mortality risk. Although great controversies flared in the past as to the relative incidence of ulcer recurrences after subtotal gastrectomy depending upon either Billroth I or Billroth II reconstructions, there does not seem to be a great difference in the present rates of ulcer recurrence between gastroduodenostomy and gastrojejunostomy.

Since the rate of ulcer recurrence is lowest with gastric resection plus truncal vagotomy, and since any *recurrent* ulcer can be assumed to represent a virulent ulcer diathesis, we perform truncal vagotomy and distal gastric resection on every patient with a recurrent ulcer, with the idea that we should give these serious ulcers the very *best* chance of cure. Therefore, if a patient has had a truncal vagotomy and drainage procedure that results in recurrent ulceration, we redo the truncal vagotomy and resect the distal stomach and do either a Billroth I or a Billroth II procedure (I prefer a Billroth I). Recurrent ulcers are usually more easily handled in patients with Billroth II anastomosis than in patients with Billroth I. Recurrent ulcers adjacent to a gastroduodenostomy frequently penetrate into the pancreas and are often difficult to manage. If someone has had a recurrent ulcer after a previous subtotal gastrectomy and vagotomy, we do a revagotomy and a re-resection. With recurrent ulcer in a patient who has had a Billroth II operation, we excise the limb of jejunum that is anastomosed to the stomach, reestablish continuity with a jejunojejunostomy, and then do another gastrojejunostomy. In patients with a recurrent ulcer after Billroth I, we usually re-resect the stomach, divide the duodenum, close the duodenal stump and do a Billroth II anastomosis. Patients with recurrent ulcers after either Billroth I or II subtotal gastrectomy should also have a truncal vagotomy.

FIG 26–4

A. In performing a revagotomy, we carefully dissect the esophageal hiatus looking for any persistent vagal fibers. The most likely source of persistent innervation is a missed posterior vagal fiber; this can often be identified by anterior traction on the cardia of the stomach. Feeling behind, a persistent vagal trunk is often seen *(arrow)* or felt, and can be divided. Some persistent vagal fibers are intramural within the esophagus. Distal traction will often reveal small, palpable cables within the muscle of the esophagus. When these small vagal fibers are cut, they pop back into the esophageal musculature.

B. In patients with a recurrent marginal ulcer after a Billroth II operation, we excise the loop of jejunum proximal and distal to the anastomosis and re-excise some of the gastric stump *(dotted lines)* so as to leave about 15% to 20% of the original gastric volume. We discard this segment, do a jejunojejunostomy, and then a regastrojejunostomy.

C. This figure shows the completed reoperative procedure with another truncal vagotomy, and re-resection of the stomach and excision of the site of the jejunal ulceration and jejunojejunostomy and regastrojejunostomy.

D. Similarly, in patients with recurrent ulcer after Billroth I resection, if the patient has had a previous vagotomy we do a revagotomy; if not, we do a truncal vagotomy. Similarly, we excise the proximal duodenum and a segment of the stomach, as shown by the *dotted line*. We then do whatever is necessary in order to manage the recurrent ulcer (see **G–N**). After this is done, we may do a closure of the lesser curvature and reanastomosis of the stomach to the duodenum. Alternatively, as shown in **E,** we may convert to a Billroth II.

E. If the decision is made to convert to a Billroth II, the duodenal stump is then closed either by suture, as shown here, or by staple, and a loop gastrojejunostomy is then created. We usually bring a short loop anterior to the transverse colon and anastomose the antimesenteric border of the jejunum to the greater curvature of the residual stomach.

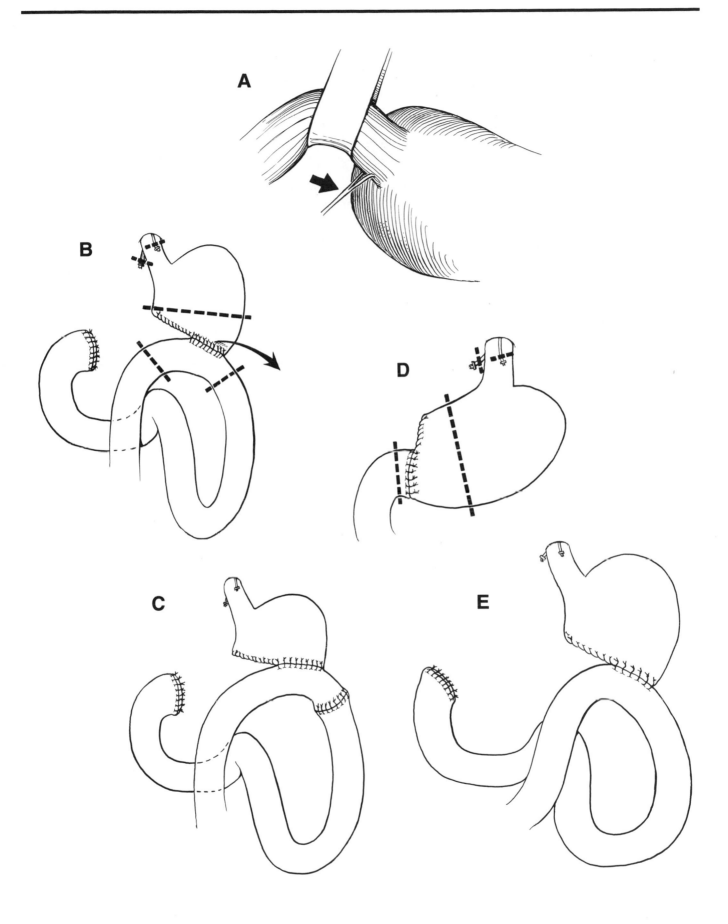

F.   This shows a recurrent ulcer in the posterior suture line in a gastroduodenal anastomosis after truncal vagotomy and antrectomy and Billroth I anastomosis. The ulcer has eroded into the superior aspect of the head of the pancreas posteriorly. In repairing this, we mobilize the distal 10 to 15 cm of the greater curvature of the stomach and about 5 to 10 cm to the lesser curvature so that we can divide the stomach and roll the distal gastric remnant distally. This resection can often be facilitated by making a distal gastrotomy so as to visualize and palpate the ulcer. The distal stomach and posterior duodenal are often badly scarred, inflamed, and edematous, and visualizing the ulcer from inside is often helpful.

G.   The descending duodenum is mobilized by a Kocher maneuver *(shaded line along descending duodenum),* and the esophageal hiatus is explored and a revagotomy performed. We divide the stomach between Payr clamps at the proximal *dotted line* and the duodenum between large Kocher clamps at the distal *dotted line.*

H.   This shows the divided duodenum, the posterior penetrating ulcer into the head of the pancreas, and the placement of sutures so as to bring the duodenum down onto the pancreas and over the ulcer for closure.

I.   This shows the duodenum closed over the ulcer crater with the Jackson-Pratt drain adjacent to the suture line.

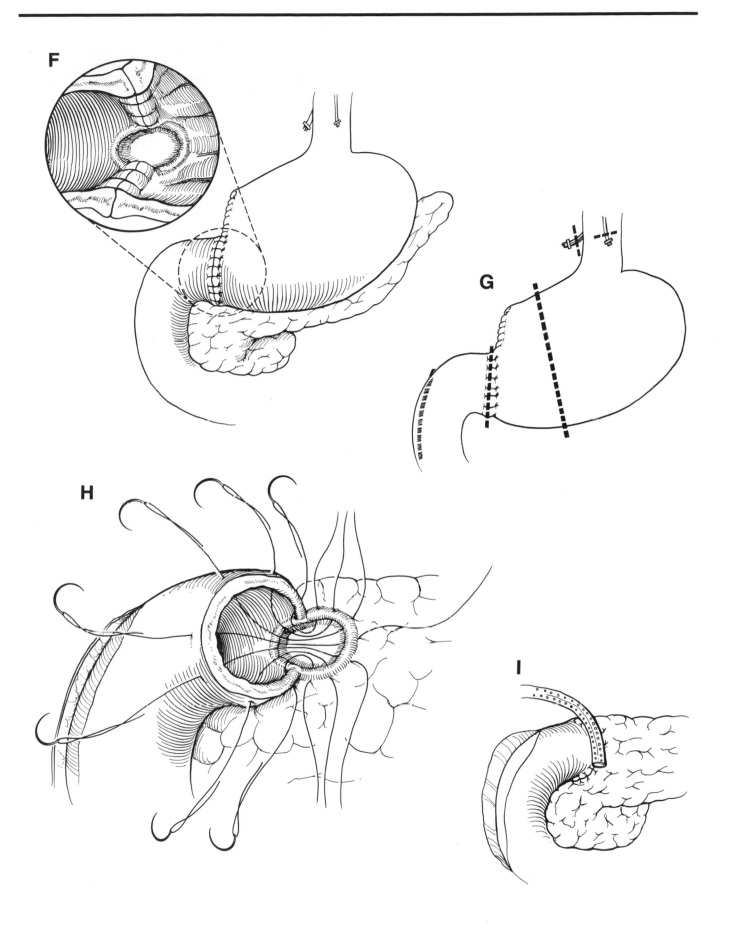

J. Another alternative (so-called Nissen III procedure) in closing a duodenal stump adjacent to a large, penetrating recurrent duodenal ulcer is to close the lumen of the duodenum itself with a running suture and, after a generous Kocher maneuver, advance the serosa of the duodenum to the left so as to cover the ulcer bed with the external wall of the duodenum. This closure is illustrated (**K–M.**)

K. The scarred wall of the penetrating ulcer is included in the closure of the duodenal lumen with a running suture.

L. After a good closure is obtained, we then advance the full-thickness wall of the duodenum so as to provide coverage of the exposed ulcer crater.

M. This closure is completed with interrupted 3-0 polyglactin (Vicryl) sutures through the wall of the rim of the ulcer crater and the full-thickness wall of the advanced duodenum. (Figures **J–M** after Jan Redden.)

N. This figure shows the completed resection with the revagotomy, the closure of the duodenum buttressed with a tab of omentum, placement of a Jackson-Pratt drain, and the new gastrojejunostomy.

J

K

L

M

J-M after Jan Redden

N

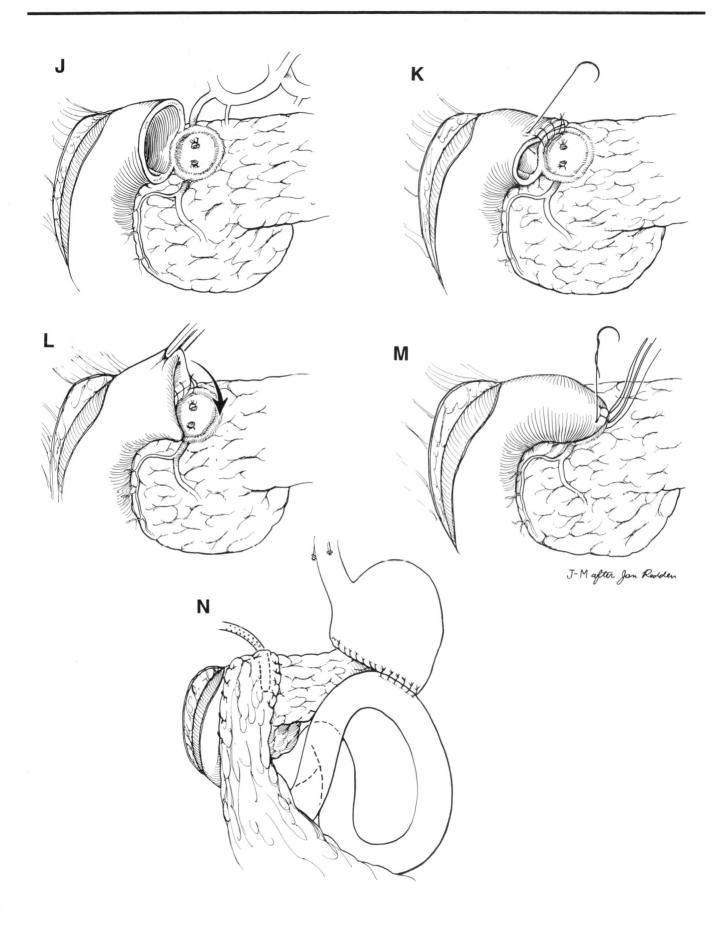

Late Complications: Alkaline Reflux Gastritis (Treated by Roux-en-Y Gastrojejunostomy)

I should first admit that I am skeptical of the diagnosis of alkaline reflux gastritis. That is not to say that the condition doesn't exist, but rather that I have a persistent skepticism as to whether it is a discrete entity that can be fixed by some operative maneuver. For decades before the term was first applied in the early 1970s, patients who had undergone subtotal gastrectomy suffered epigastric distress and occasional bilious vomiting, the most likely etiology of which was a misplanned or misexecuted primary operation. Once the diagnosis "alkaline reflux gastritis" was announced, hundreds of patients were discovered and subjected to Roux-en-Y gastrojejunostomy. Many of these patients got better, but it was difficult to discount the placebo effects, since no appropriate control studies were carried out. The problem with a Roux-en-Y gastrojejunostomy is that it is potentially an ulcerogenic procedure and its use in this instance led, inevitably, to its application as a *primary* anastomosis for patients who had subtotal gastrectomy for duodenal ulcer disease. (The recurrence rate of peptic ulceration in these patients has been extraordinarily high.) Peptic ulceration after Roux-en-Y operation for patients with postoperative alkaline reflux gastritis has certainly occurred, but the incidence is low because the gastritis has destroyed most of the parietal cells. With time, however, if the operation is sufficiently successful so that the gastritis heals, the parietal cells will regrow and we should see a fair number of these patients coming in with marginal ulcerations. There is no doubt but that several patients, incapacitated by pain and bilious vomiting, have initially done well after Roux-en-Y gastrojejunostomy diverted bile from the stomach. The illustrations below depict steps in the operation.

FIG 26–5

A. This illustrates division of the jejunal loop in a patient with a subtotal gastrectomy and gastrojejunostomy. The jejunum is divided immediately proximal to the gastrojejunostomy with a GIA stapling device. This diverts the flow of bile and pancreatic juice away from the gastrojejunal stoma. It also, of course, removes the protection of alkaline bile and alkaline pancreatic secretions from the jejunal mucosa and leaves it to the unbuffered mercy of acid-gastric juice.

B. The Roux-en-Y is completed by performance of an end-to-side jejunojejunostomy 50 to 60 cm distal to the gastrojejunostomy so as to prevent reflux of bile into the stomach. The jejunojejunostomy can be performed either by hand, as shown here, or by use of the stapling device (**Fig 25–1, L,** p. 161).

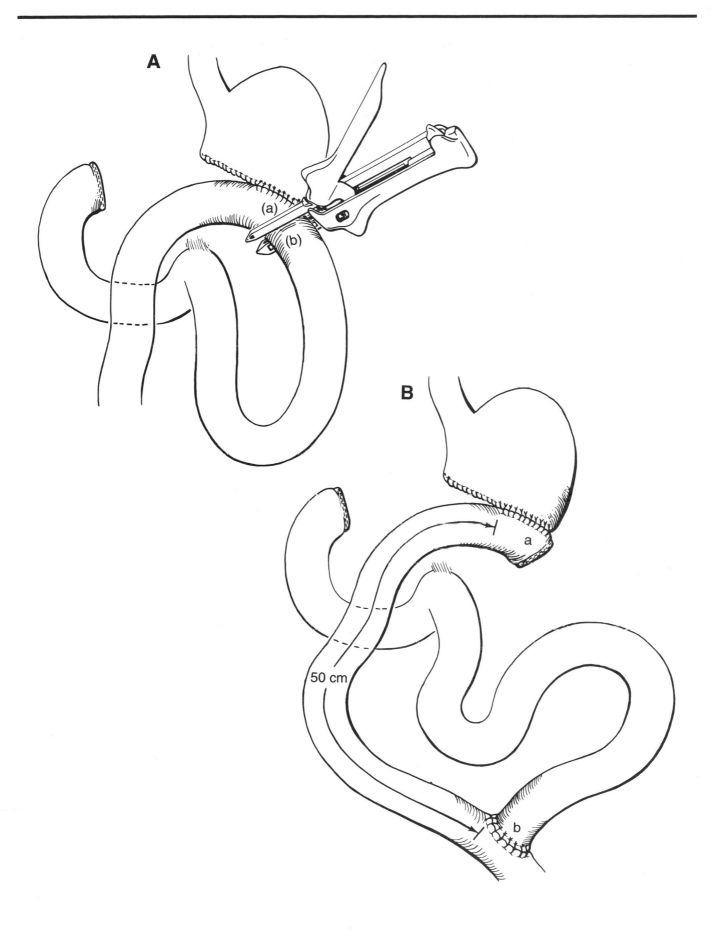

27

Operative Removal of Foreign Objects From the Stomach

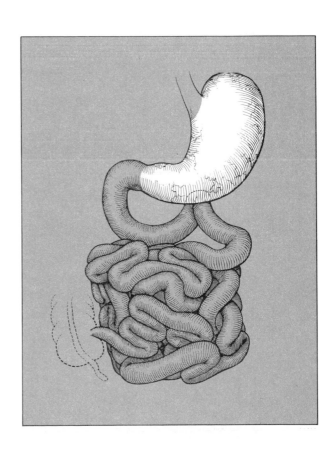

Babies and young children ingest coins and pins accidentally; psychotic patients may ingest almost anything, either accidentally or as part of an established pattern of behavior. Many foreign bodies will traverse the gut and be passed in the stool without incident. Other foreign bodies can be removed from the stomach by endoscopic manipulation without great incident. The problem is when to operate. Each case, of course, must be decided individually. Pediatricians with great experience are often fairly blasé, and will patiently wait for long periods; they have as a maxim, the concept that anything that passes the pylorus will probably pass on through the anus. When following up someone who has a radiopaque foreign body in the stomach that may be able to pass, there will be a great temptation to obtain radiographs with great frequency, most of which will, in retrospect, be useless. Any object with sharp edges can lacerate the mucosa and cause bleeding. Often it is best simply to fix a deadline and plan to operate if the object has not passed. Clearly some objects that are large or that have sharp edges will require operative removal. Before operating, the stomach should be emptied as well as possible by nasogastric suction. The foreign object should be localized by endoscopy or by radiography. The surgeon should not be surprised if the object is somewhere else in the stomach, or beyond, at operation.

Bezoars are long-standing concretions occasionally found in the stomach or small bowel. They are of three types, according to their composition: phytobezoars (fruit and vegetable), trichobezoars (hair balls), or a mixture of the two. The juice of unripe persimmons forms a shellac-like resin in the acid lumen of the stomach and is responsible for many phytobezoars. Some patients are addicted to unripe persimmons and may repeatedly require bezoar extractions. Patients with gastric outlets narrowed by peptic or postoperative scarring are predisposed to the development of bezoars. One of the finest medical reviews of any subject, in my opinion, was compiled on the subject of bezoars by DeBakey when he was a house officer (DeBakey M, Ochsner A: Bezoars and concretions: Comprehensive review of literature with analysis of 303 collected cases and presentation of 8 additional cases. *Surgery* 1938; 4:934, and 1939; 5:132). Most bezoars can be managed by endoscopic break-up and extraction, especially after treatment with papain (the active ingredient in Adolph's Meat Tenderizer, which may be used). Some large bezoars may require operative extraction.

FIG 27–1

A. At operation for foreign bodies retained in the stomach. The stomach should be opened by means of a transverse gastrotomy, usually performed in the distal stomach unless the object is fixed somewhere else.

B. Stay sutures are placed in the gastrotomy wound and the wound inspected. Sometimes a foreign body almost leaps out of the wound and sometimes prolonged searches are required. When the object is removed, we insert retractors and carefully inspect the mucosa. On occasion we will find lacerations that are bleeding. These can be handled by a simple suture.

C. The wound is closed first with a Connell suture through all layers, which is then reinforced with interrupted 4-0 polyglactin (Vicryl) sutures.

D. Some patients present major problems. This abdominal film is from a retarded person who had been operated upon four times previously for removal of massive metallic foreign bodies. This radiograph shows that what is apparently a bullet and a safety pin-like object have passed the stomach, whereas a large number of radiopaque foreign bodies remain in the stomach. At gastrotomy he was found not only to have all of these metallic objects but also half of a tennis shoe.

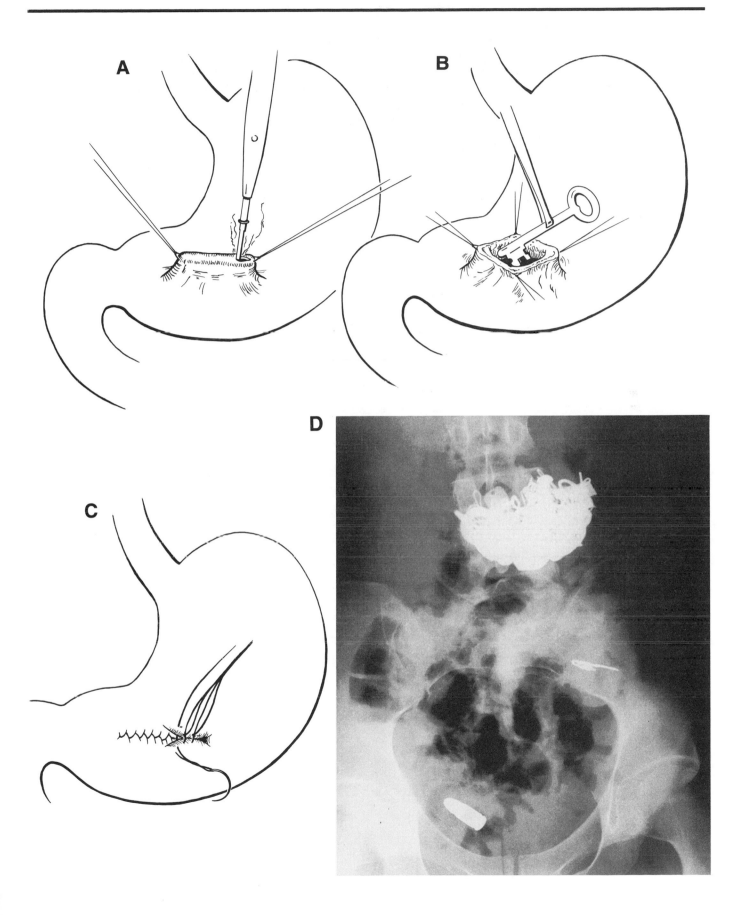

E. Most small bezoars can be extracted endoscopically after breaking them apart with endoscopic forceps. Bezoars can often be softened by instillation of solutions of papain, which should be allowed to stay in situ for several hours. Some patients develop severe reactions to papain, so small test doses should be applied initially.

F. If the bezoar cannot be removed endoscopically, operative removal is necessary. The inlying mass should be palpated and an incision (made sufficiently large to allow easy extraction) should be made through the wall of the stomach.

G. The mass of vegetable fibers or hair or both should be taken out of the stomach, and any bezoar material that has escaped into the duodenum should be milked back into the stomach. The stomach may be achlorhydric and the material in the bezoar may be contaminated, so care should be taken to avoid peritoneal contamination.

H. The stomach should be closed in two layers. Before this, the entire bowel should be inspected to rule out the possibility of bezoar material having passed the pylorus. Anything that passes the pylorus will almost certainly pass through the rest of the gut, but early resumption of gut function might be facilitated by milking the material back into the stomach for extraction, or into the colon.

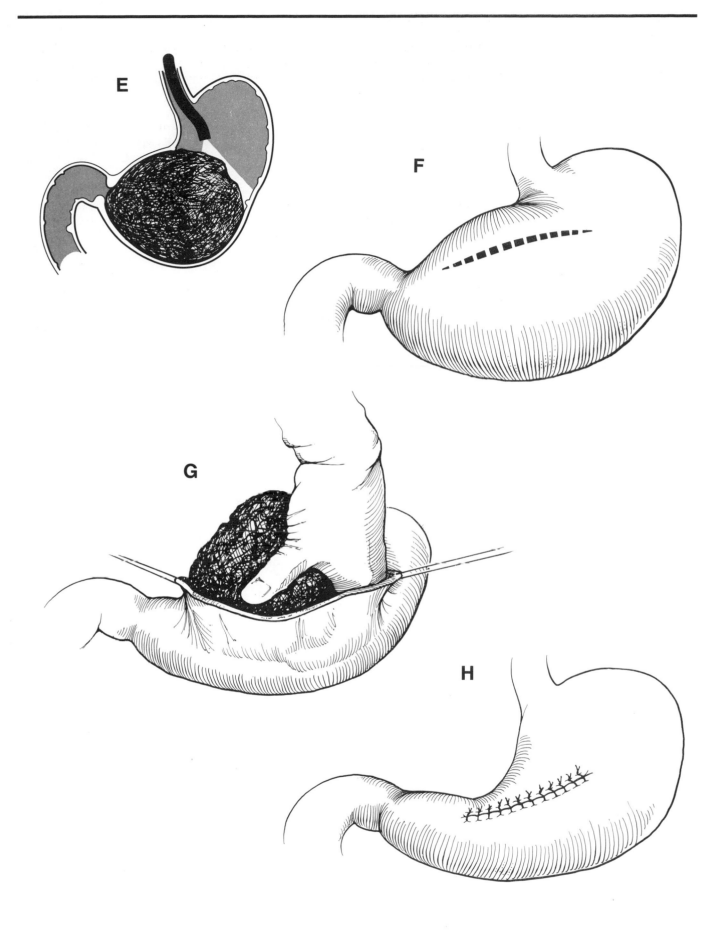

DUODENUM

Part II

The reader is reminded that operative procedures on the duodenum for duodenal ulcer disease are included under "Stomach" (Section I), since peptic ulcer disease is shared by the stomach and duodenum. We have included in this section a discussion and a depiction of radical pancreaticoduodenectomy (Whipple procedure) in the management of cancer of the papilla of Vater or of the duodenum itself.

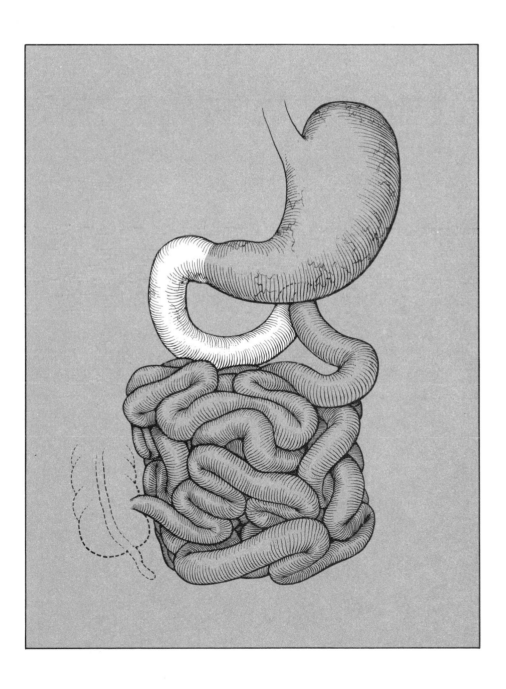

Anatomy
of the Duodenum

28

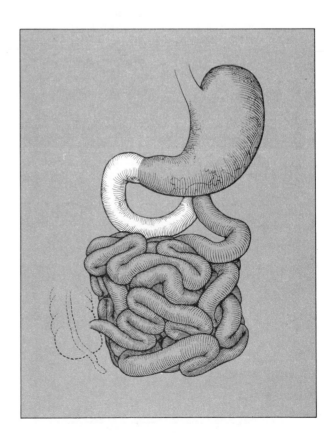

The term *duodenum* comes from the Latin word meaning twelve, a reference to its supposed length of 12 fingerbreadths. Embryologically, the duodenum is that part of the foregut just beyond the stomach, which, during the period of foregut rotation, ends up with its first portion of the duodenum to the right of the midline at about the T12–L1 interspace, and its junction with the jejunum just to the left of the second lumbar vertebra. Except for the proximal bulb, the duodenum is retroperitoneal.

FIG 28–1

A. The duodenum is divided into four portions: superior *(I)*, descending *(II)*, transverse *(III)*, and ascending *(IV)*. Nearly all of the first portion is occupied by the slightly dilated duodenal bulb whose mucosa is characterized by a lack of folds. The characteristic circular folds of small bowel mucosa begin just before the end of the first portion of the duodenum, and they extend throughout the small bowel. These circular folds (also called *plicae circulares of Kerckring* or *valvulae conniventes*) provide a great increase in small-bowel mucosal surface area; folds are abundant in the duodenum and jejunum and become less prominent in the ileum. The common bile duct enters the pancreas immediately posterior to the duodenal bulb, and runs within the head of the pancreas for its most distal 3 to 4 cm. The common bile duct and the main pancreatic duct open together onto the medial wall of the midportion of the second part of the duodenum at the duodenal papilla (ampulla of Vater). The first, second, and third portions of the duodenum constitute the C-loop, in the concavity of which lies the head of the pancreas. The superior mesenteric vessels emerge from behind the pancreas to cross over the third part of the duodenum. The fourth segment of the duodenum ascends to the duodenojejunal flexure, which is suspended from the posterior body wall by the ligament of Treitz. In order to visualize the distal second portion or the proximal third portion of the duodenum, the hepatic flexure of the colon must be mobilized so as to lift the attachment of the transverse mesocolon away from the posterior body wall, affording access to the duodenum. The distal third and the fourth portion of the duodenum can be approached by mobilizing the retroperitoneal attachments of the left side of the transverse mesocolon. One may, of course, take down the entire transverse mesocolon, taking care to avoid injury to the middle colic vessels or to the common alternate origin of the common hepatic or right hepatic artery from the middle colic artery. Injuries to the retroperitoneal duodenum are often complicated by retroperitoneal hematomas that obscure the anatomy. One way to manage this is to follow the visible and palpable duodenum itself, adhering closely to the anterior wall. This approach is applicable when coming from either right or left, bearing in mind that the inferior mesenteric vein joins the splenic vein just behind the duodenojejunal flexure, and also keeping in mind the position of the superior mesenteric artery and vein as they go over the third part of the duodenum. The superior mesenteric artery gives off the middle colic artery as its first branch and the middle colic artery ascends in the transverse mesocolon at about the level of the duodenojejunal flexure.

A

I

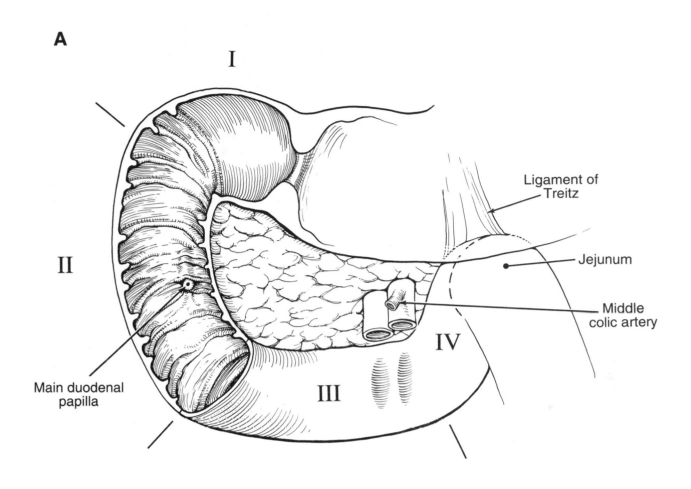

II

Ligament of
Treitz

Jejunum

Middle
colic artery

IV

III

Main duodenal
papilla

B. The duodenum shares much of its blood supply with the pancreas. The gastroduodenal branch of the hepatic artery (from the celiac trunk) goes behind the duodenal bulb. Behind the bulb, the gastroduodenal artery may receive a collateral from the transverse pancreatic artery (shown but not labeled), which may cause troublesome rebleeding after suture-ligation of a bleeding duodenal ulcer (see U-Stitch, Chapter 17; pp. 110 and 111). At the inferior margin of the bulb, the gastroduodenal artery divides into a right gastroepiploic branch and a superior pancreaticoduodenal branch. The right gastroepiploic supplies the distal greater curvature of the stomach and the right side of the gastrocolic ligament. The superior pancreaticoduodenal artery supplies branches to the proximal duodenum and head of the pancreas and anastomoses freely with the inferior pancreaticoduodenal branch of the superior mesenteric so as to supply blood to the third and fourth parts of the duodenum and head and neck of the pancreas. Both the superior and inferior pancreaticoduodenal arteries are actually divided into anterior and posterior arcades, not shown here.

C. The small bowel emerges from its retroperitoneal position at the duodenojejunal flexure, and the entire jejunoileum is an intraperitoneal organ lying below the transverse mesocolon, suspended from the posterior body wall by the oblique (downwards and to the right) attachment of the small bowel mesentery. At the site of emergence of the jejunum, there are often small potential spaces above, lateral to, and below the left margin of the duodenojejunal flexure. These spaces, called, respectively, *a,* the superior duodenal fossa, *b,* the paraduodenal fossa, or *c,* the inferior duodenal fossa, may be the site of internal herniation of the small bowel, a rare cause of small bowel obstruction. Anyone who makes the preoperative diagnosis of an internal hernia into a duodenal fossa deserves instant stardom, but the possibility should certainly be borne in mind when operating on patients who develop small bowel obstruction and who have no peritoneal adhesive bands, abdominal wall hernias or tumors, or areas of bowel ischemia. Occasionally, the internal hernia may contain a trapped loop of bowel, and be surprisingly large. Once the hernia is reduced, the fossa should be obliterated by dividing and excising the overlying peritoneum. Management of the herniated bowel will depend upon whether its blood supply has been compromised.

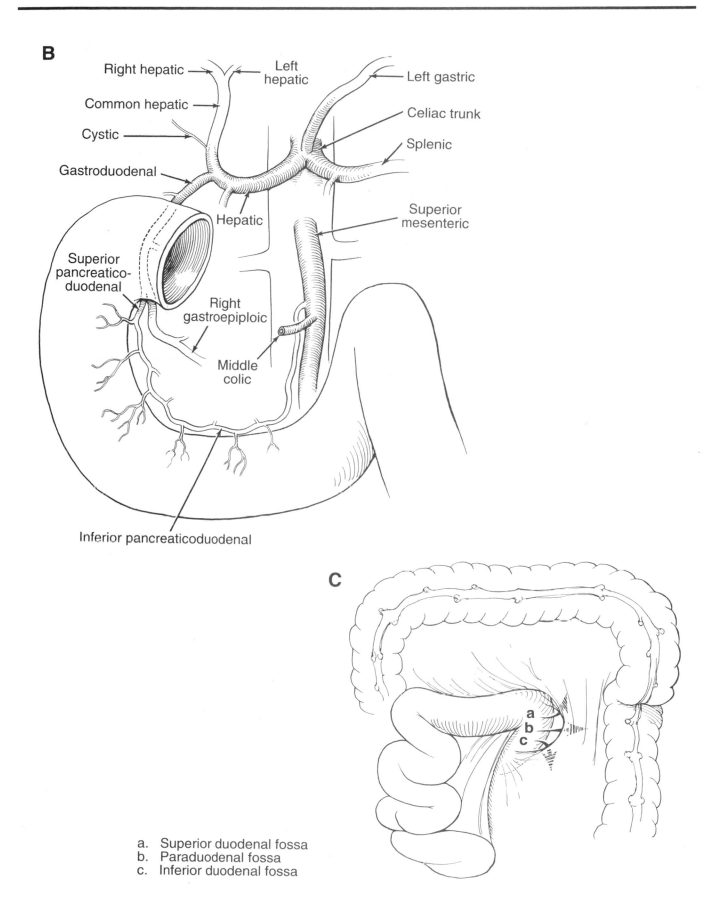

B

Right hepatic

Left hepatic

Left gastric

Common hepatic

Celiac trunk

Cystic

Splenic

Gastroduodenal

Hepatic

Superior
mesenteric

Superior
pancreatico-
duodenal

Right
gastroepiploic

Middle
colic

Inferior pancreaticoduodenal

C

a. Superior duodenal fossa
b. Paraduodenal fossa
c. Inferior duodenal fossa

Duodenal Obstruction in the Newborn

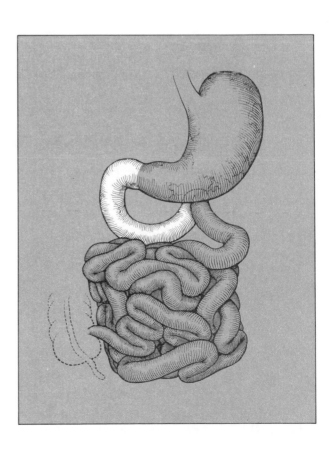

29

Atresia or Annular Pancreas

Bilious vomiting in the newborn always constitutes a serious situation, since nearly all the causes are potentially lethal. The three most common causes are atresia of the duodenum or proximal small bowel, annular pancreas, or midgut volvulus. Since midgut volvulus threatens infarction of the entire small intestine, early diagnosis is essential. Bile in the vomitus signals a site of obstruction distal to the papilla of Vater. A plain x-ray ("babygram") will show the classic double-bubble sign of a dilated stomach and a dilated proximal duodenum, if the site of obstruction is caused by duodenal atresia or annular pancreas. A rare cause of duodenal obstruction is a web or wind-sock diaphragm, which may also cause the radiologic double bubble. The web is treated by anastomosis of the proximal obstructed duodenum to the duodenum distal to the obstruction, if feasible, or to the jejunum. If there is no double-bubble sign, instillation of contrast may show that the second part of the duodenum maintains a straight course downward and does not have a horizontal third portion crossing the midline. This straight downward descent of the third part of the duodenum is a clue to malrotation, and midgut volvulus is a strong possibility. Retroperitoneal bands (Ladd's bands) are often associated with failure of rotation, and they may obstruct the duodenum itself. Since the envelopment of the duodenum by a ring of pancreas deposited during rotation of the foregut will suppress further development of the duodenum, annular pancreas and duodenal atresia bring about identical pathologic results. They can be treated identically, that is, by anastomosis of the proximal dilated duodenum to a loop of proximal, collapsed jejunum. Many pediatric surgeons now prefer an anastomosis between the proximal obstructed duodenum and the duodenum distal to the obstruction (for all forms of congenital duodenal obstruction).

FIG 29–1

A. In intrauterine life, the ventral anlage of the pancreas grows into the ventral mesentery of the foregut and the dorsal anlage into the dorsal mesentery. When the foregut rotates, ordinarily the ventral anlage rotates 180 degrees around the second part of the duodenum so as to form the head of the pancreas, and the dorsal anlage lies against the posterior body wall to form the body and tail. Rarely, fragments of pancreatic tissue are shed during this hejira so as to form a ring of pancreatic tissue that compresses the second part of the duodenum and prevents further development during fetal growth. Small pancreatic rests (fragments of pancreatic tissue shed during the rotation) may appear throughout the upper abdomen. Annular pancreas usually causes duodenal obstruction in the newborn; rarely, obstruction may not be manifest until later life. I cared for one man who grew to young adulthood before his duodenum became obstructed. Division of the ring of pancreatic tissue is useless and dangerous: useless because the underlying duodenum is severely stenotic or even atretic, and dangerous because there may be a pancreatic duct within the annulus. Correction involves an anastomosis between the proximal obstructed duodenum and the distal collapsed bowel.

B. Duodenal atresia usually occurs distal to the papilla and is caused by whatever brings about intrauterine atresia of segments of the gut (thought to be periods of unexplained ischemia).

C. The treatment we use is a one-layer side-by-side anastomosis between the first part of the duodenum and the distal duodenum or proximal jejunum. The lumen of the distal bowel is often small and the discrepancy in size is great. The lumen of the bowel can be enlarged by inserting a needle between occluding noncrushing clamps and instilling normal saline under slight pressure.

D. Most surgeons now utilize a single-layer anastomosis, especially if the discrepancy in lumens is great. This shows the completed repair.

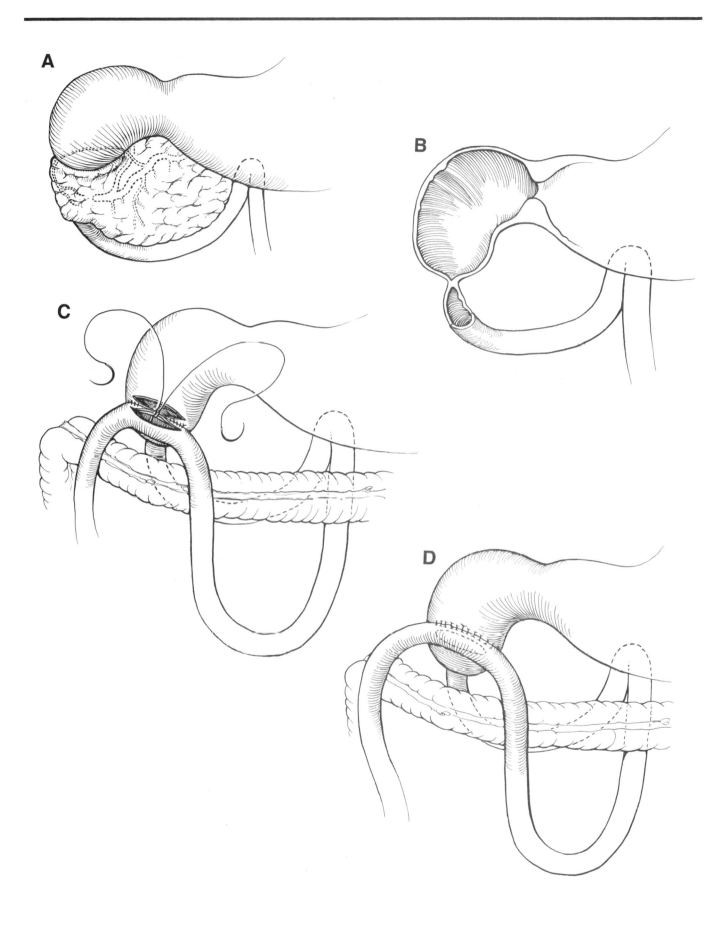

E. This shows the alternate, and now probably preferred method of correction, which involves mobilization of the third part of the duodenum to allow a duodenoduodenostomy. Note the Kochner maneuver used to mobilize the proximal duodenum.

F. The side-to-side stoma should be made as large as possible.

G. This figure gives an approximation of the relative frequency of congenital atresia of various segments of the bowel.

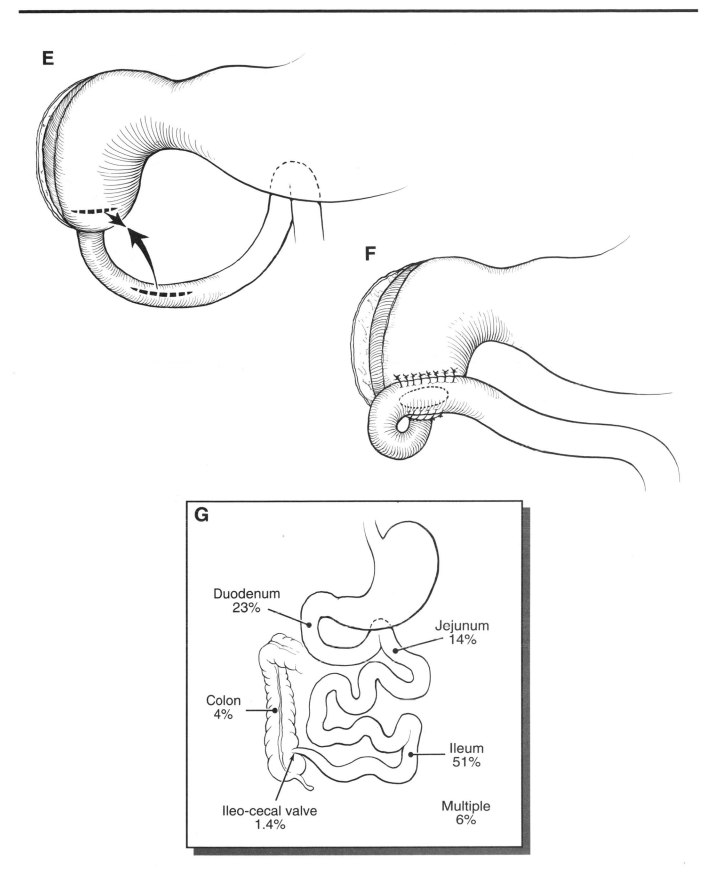

E

F

G

Duodenum
23%

Jejunum
14%

Colon
4%

Ileum
51%

Ileo-cecal valve
1.4%

Multiple
6%

Midgut Volvulus or Ladd's Bands

Bilious vomiting in the newborn denotes trouble. The cause can be duodenal atresia or an annular pancreas (both of which obstruct the duodenum), or midgut volvulus, itself caused by failure of complete bowel rotation. In patients with duodenal obstruction, a plain abdominal film will show the double-bubble sign. If that is absent, instillation of opaque material may show flow of contrast in a straight inferior path from the second part of the duodenum into the midgut volvulus. Individuals with incomplete rotation of the gut may also have complete or incomplete obstruction of the distal duodenum caused by transverse attachment of an abnormal mesentery, partially suspending the malrotated bowel. This mesentery, so-called Ladd's bands, suspends the proximal colon from the right posterior abdominal wall and in crossing over the duodenum may obstruct it. Obstruction by Ladd's bands often accompanies midgut volvulus, but each may occur without the other. Patients with midgut volvulus may undergo operative reduction of the volvulus, and if the bands are not divided, the duodenum may later be obstructed by them. Some patients develop duodenal obstruction from Ladd's bands in later life, without midgut volvulus. The important thing, of course, is that response to bilious vomiting must be prompt and certain. If the patient does have midgut volvulus, the bowel can infarct within a very short time, often leaving insufficient bowel for maintenance of life. Infarction usually affects the bowel from the distal duodenum to the midtransverse colon. As is clear from the illustrations below, patients who have Ladd's bands obstructing the duodenum along with midgut volvulus may present with a radiographic picture of duodenal obstruction.

FIG 29–2

A. The illustration depicts failure of complete rotation with midgut volvulus, as well as duodenal obstruction due to Ladd's bands. The bowel should be immediately untwisted, almost always best effected by counterclockwise rotation, as shown. Any dead bowel should be excised. Bowel of questionable viability is best handled by a second look 12 to 16 hours later. If the entire bowel is infarcted, many surgeons do nothing to the bowel.

B. If the bowel is viable after detorsion, the duodenum should be carefully inspected and any peritoneal bands crossing it should be divided.

C. No attempt should be made to rearrange the bowel into a normal configuration. The duodenum should be allowed to run straight downward into the jejunoileum and if the entire colon is on the left side, it should remain there. The entire bowel should be inspected for possible atresia or other additional causes of obstruction.

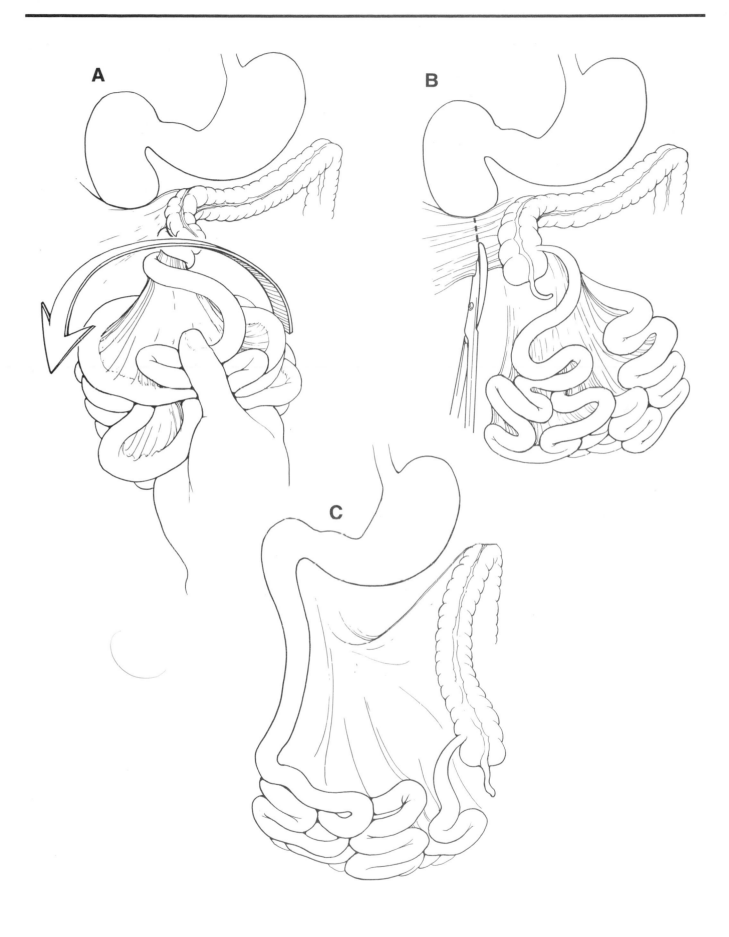

A

B

C

Duodenal Diverticular Disease

30

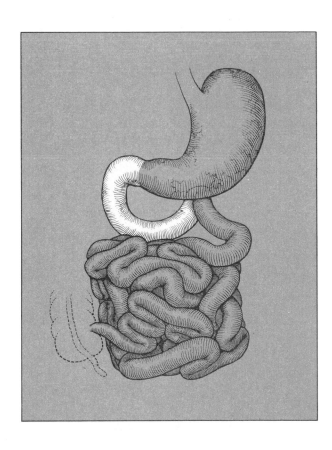

Diverticula occur throughout the entire gut, excluding only the rectum. Usually the diverticula consist of outpouchings of mucosa protruding through the muscle wall. If the diverticulum occurs in the portion of the gut covered by peritoneum, it will have a serosal coat, but if the diverticulum is retroperitoneal, it will consist, usually, only of mucosa. Full-thickness diverticula may occur rarely when inflammatory or neoplastic adhesions exert traction on a small segment of bowel and create what is probably best termed a false diverticulum. Diverticula of the stomach are rare and when present cause trouble only infrequently. They can either be divided with clamps at the base, oversewn, and the stump inverted into the stomach, or they can be inverted entirely into the lumen of the stomach, clamped, severed, and repaired from the inside. Duodenal diverticula, on the other hand, are common (next to the colon, the duodenum is the most common site of diverticulum formation). Duodenal diverticula are rare in persons under the age of 25 years but above the age of 50 years their incidence increases greatly; it has been estimated in different series to be as high as 5% to 20% of all people more than 50 years of age. The vast majority of duodenal diverticula are asymptomatic, and if an asymptomatic diverticulum is found on upper GI series or endoscopy or at operation, it should probably be ignored (unless it is physically in the way of some other needed operative procedure). Occasionally duodenal diverticula will bleed or perforate or, rarely, obstruct the duodenum. The rare periampullary duodenal diverticulum may become filled with dietary detritus and exert pressure on the common bile duct and may cause jaundice and, rarely, cholangitis. It is important not to extend indications for operation to include people with unexplained abdominal pain. Nor should retention of barium within diverticula serve by itself as any indication for operation. The important message is that the great majority of diverticula cause no trouble. We operate only on those that cause serious symptoms. Exposure of the diverticula may be simple or vastly difficult. Careful preoperative endoscopic and barium studies will often be of great help in their localization. If the diverticulum protrudes into the peritoneal cavity, localization is usually simple, but protrusion of diverticula of the second part of the duodenum into the retroperitoneal space or into the area between the pancreas and duodenum often makes exposure difficult. Localization may sometimes be facilitated by placing noncrushing clamps proximally and distally and distending the duodenal loop with air or water. Diverticulectomy is usually simple: the diverticulum may be inverted into the lumen, clamped, and amputated at its base and the pedicle oversewn. A similar procedure of amputation and oversewing may be used to remove a diverticulum on the outside of the duodenum. If the site of protrusion is retroperitoneal, great care should be taken in closing the duodenum, since there is no serosa. The principle that guides excision of periampullary diverticula, of course, is to remove the diverticulum without injury to the bile or pancreatic ducts.

FIG 30–1

A. Distribution of duodenal diverticula appears to be random. Many surgeons believe that diverticula of the second part of the duodenum are more likely to cause trouble, but this may simply be because these diverticula are the most difficult to remove.

B. If the diverticulum is clearly visible, it can be mobilized and traction exerted on a suture in the apex. A Kocher clamp can be placed at the base and the diverticulum excised.

C. We usually close the diverticulum by placing a running 4-0 swaged polyglactin (Vicryl) suture back and forth behind the clamp in a basting stitch. We then invert that suture line with a role of interrupted 4-0 polyglactin sutures, as shown.

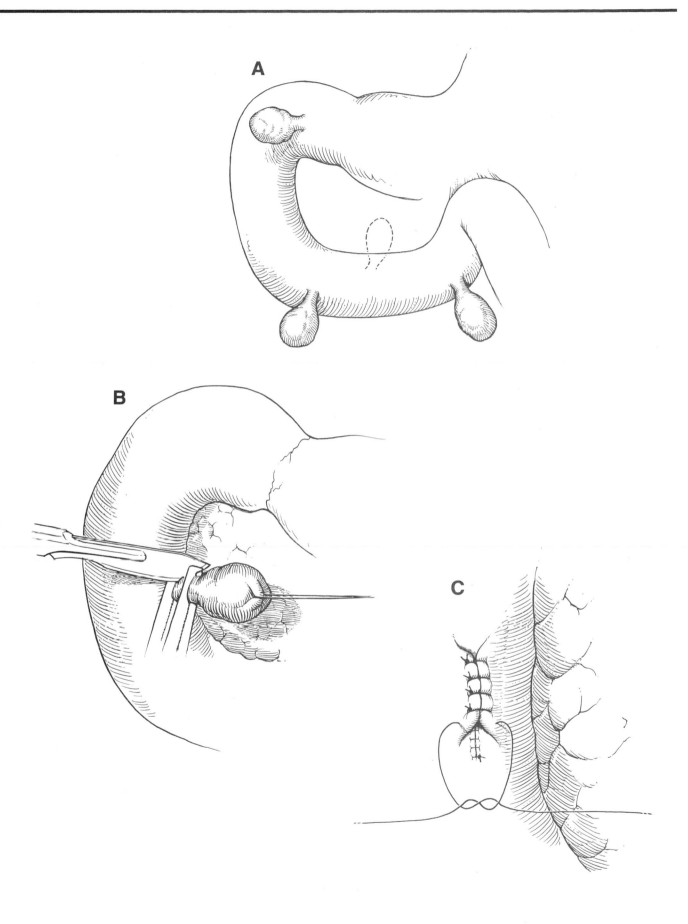

D.   If there is any possibility whatsoever that the mouth of the diverticulum may be adjacent to the papilla of Vater, the duodenum should be opened and the base exposed. This illustration shows a diverticulum protruding into the head of the pancreas (or perhaps, posterior to the head of the pancreas) and the vertical duodenal incision used to expose it.

E.   Once the aperture of the diverticulum is exposed, it is usually possible to insert a clamp, grasp the apex of the diverticulum, and invert it into the duodenal lumen. If the diverticulum is adherent, it may be necessary to mobilize the duodenum to free up the wall of the diverticulum.

F.   This shows the diverticulum fully inverted into the lumen. We place Kocher clamps at the base, put interrupted sutures deep to the deep clamp, and excise the diverticulum.

G.   The sutures are tied, thereby closing the defect.

H.   The duodenotomy may be closed either vertically or transversely. If small bites are taken, it is usually possible to close the vertical duodenotomy wound in a vertical fashion without significant narrowing of the lumen. We use two running 4-0 polyglactin swaged sutures applied in the Connell fashion.

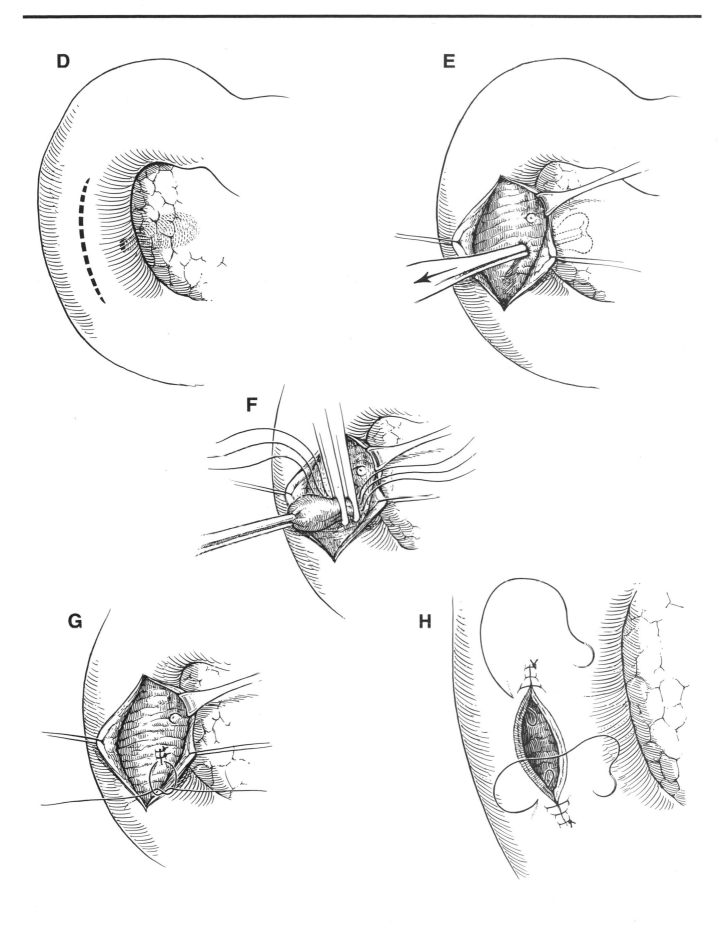

I. Figures **I–N** are devoted to the management of those unusual duodenal diverticula that appear in the periampullary location. This shows the importance of preoperative endoscopy in order to determine the site of the diverticular orifice adjacent to the papilla. Preknowledge will allow the surgeon to prepare properly. If, for some reason, the diagnosis is not made preoperatively, the site of the orifice of the diverticulum must be carefully sought, and if found in this or a similar periampullary position, it should be excised with care so as to avoid injury to the sphincter of Oddi, or bile or pancreatic ducts. A tube stent should be placed into the common bile duct and passed distally into the duodenum so as to facilitate identification and later dissection of the sphincter of Oddi.

J. A vein retractor has been placed in the diverticular orifice. The *heavy dotted line* shows the site for a circumferential periampullary incision so as to free up the papilla and sphincter. Dissection is facilitated by the presence of the plastic stent.

K. A forceps is then inserted into the diverticulum and the tip of the diverticulum is grasped.

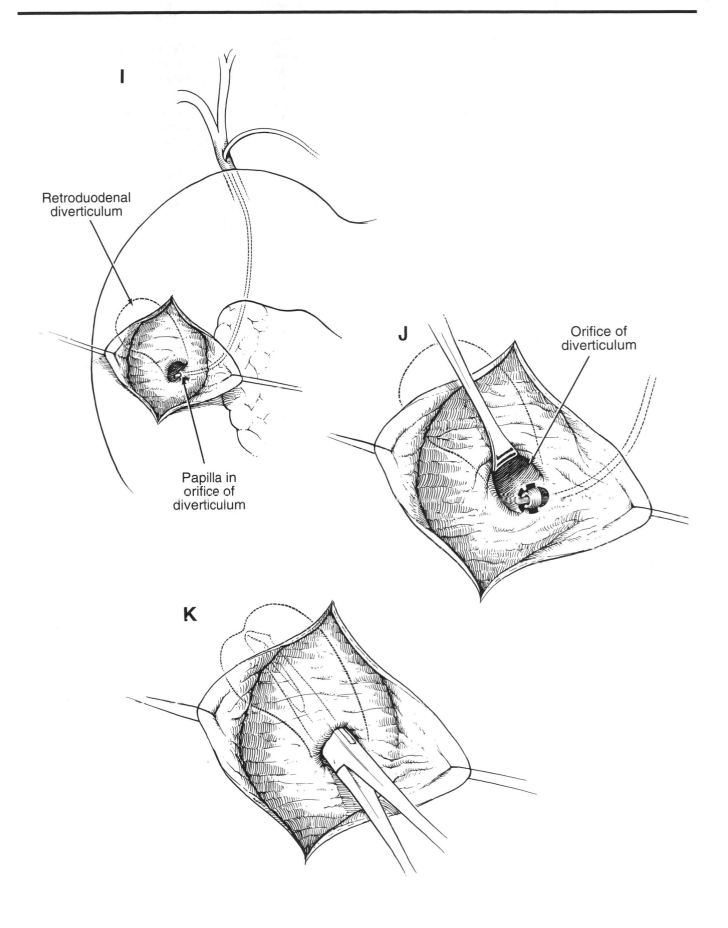

I

Retroduodenal
diverticulum

Papilla in
orifice of
diverticulum

J

Orifice of
diverticulum

K

L. The diverticulum is inverted into the lumen of the duodenum. The round opening in the wall of the base of the diverticulum is the site at which the ampullary structures were freed by a circumferential incision. The *dotted line* shows the line of division of the base of the diverticulum, which is accomplished by free-hand dissection.

M. After the diverticulum has been removed, the stent and enveloping papilla are protruded into the defect left by the division of the base of the diverticulum. The mucosa and muscle wall of the papilla are then sewn circumferentially to the wall of the duodenum.

N. This shows the completed repair of the posterior wall of the duodenum with reattachment of the papilla to the posterior wall of the duodenum and vertical closure of the remainder of the defect caused by amputation of the diverticulum. The anterior duodenotomy wound is then closed with a running 4-0 polyglactin suture placed in the Connell fashion, plus an interrupted row of 4-0 polyglactin sutures.

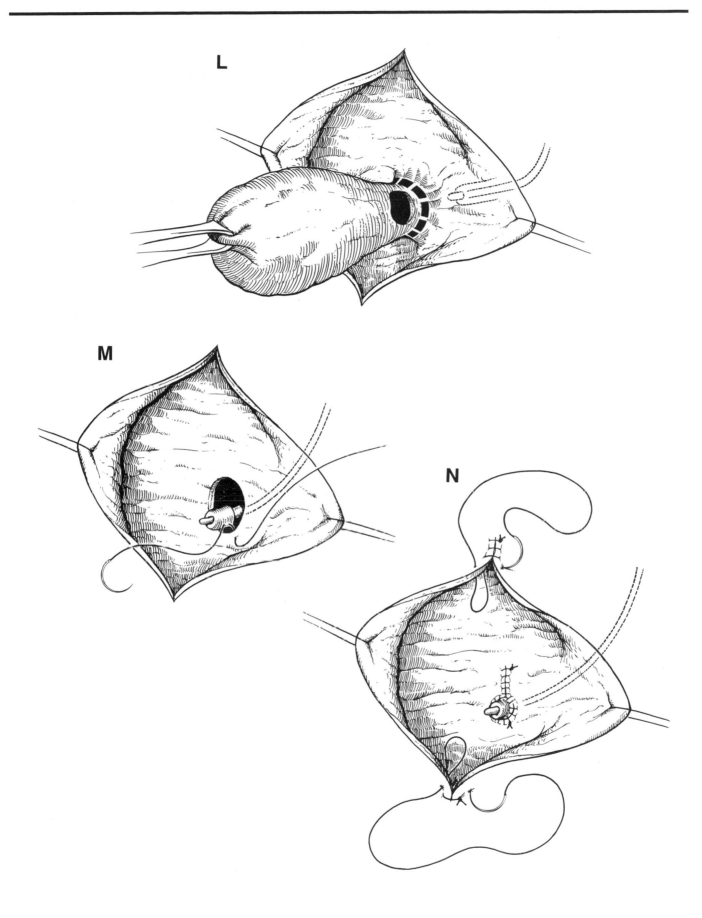

Duodenal Trauma

31

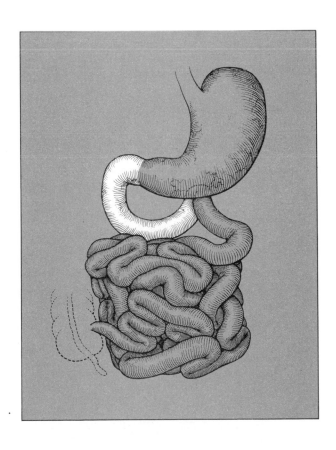

The duodenum may be injured by penetrating or blunt trauma. It is, of course, in close proximity to other vital structures (pancreas, common bile duct, liver, gallbladder, vena cava, portal vein, superior mesenteric vessels, right adrenal, and colon) so that multiple organ injury is the rule rather than the exception. Combined injuries of the duodenum and pancreas are particularly common and often present problems that are difficult to solve. Resection is rarely the answer and emergency pancreaticoduodenectomy has a near-prohibitive mortality and has almost been abandoned. If the injury is sufficiently severe, however, the surgeon should of course take whatever steps are necessary, including Whipple resection.

Vast experience with combined severe injuries at major trauma centers in America has led to a general policy of conservatism, that is, trying to patch things up, divert the enteric stream, and suppress secretions. There is no stereotypic operation for repair of duodenal injury; the surgeon must be familiar with multiple options and choose whatever seems most appropriate at the time of operation. I will present several options with a general concept of when they are indicated.

Operative priorities are the same as ever—at the very first, bleeding should be stopped and enteric leaks temporarily sealed, and the patient's blood volume restored if necessary. The surgeon should be particularly alert to occult injuries to other structures. If there is any question at all, the entire duodenum should be explored and carefully inspected along with adjacent structures. Diagnosis is sometimes difficult and retroperitoneal rupture of the duodenum from blunt trauma may be particularly vexing. We cared for a man several years ago who had been repeatedly kicked in the abdomen and back who came in with hematomas of his abdominal wall muscles. He refused admission and returned in three days with severe upper abdominal pain. Although his vital signs were stable, he was clearly quite sick and serial plain films of the abdomen eventually revealed retroperitoneal streaks of air. When we operated on him we found that his upper abdomen contained several hematomas, but not until we performed a wide Kocher maneuver and found bile staining of the retroperitoneum was it clear that he had a linear tear in the posterior wall of the descending duodenum.

Suction drainage is of great help after conservative repair; we place suction drains adjacent to the duodenal suture line and to areas of pancreatic disruption. Although all dead tissue should obviously be debrided, it is important to conserve as much duodenal tissue as possible, if attempt is to be made at primary closure. If the wound is too large for such a maneuver, we can apply a serosal patch to the wound or anastomose it to a Roux-en-Y limb of jejunum.

Exposure is vital and the surgeon operating upon patients with duodenal injuries should be familiar with techniques of exposure of all parts of the duodenum. Postoperative use of long-acting somatostatin may be of great help in suppressing gastric and pancreatic secretions.

Exposure

FIG 31–1

A. Exposure of the descending duodenum can be accomplished by means of a Kocher maneuver. This illustration shows a through-and-through gunshot wound of the lateral wall of the descending duodenum. The peritoneum has been incised so as to allow medial retraction of the descending duodenum.

B. Medial retraction of the descending duodenum reveals the posterior surface of the head of the pancreas and the underlying vena cava. The hematoma shown here on the right was caused by injury to a small tributary to the inferior vena cava, which was ligated. The vena cava itself was intact. The posterior wound of exit of the missile is clearly shown. In this instance, we excised both the wound of entrance and of exit by cutting along the dotted line.

C. We closed the resultant defect in two layers, the first a continuous running Connell suture of 4-0 polyglactin (Vicryl), which was then inverted with a interrupted row of 4-0 polyglactin sutures.

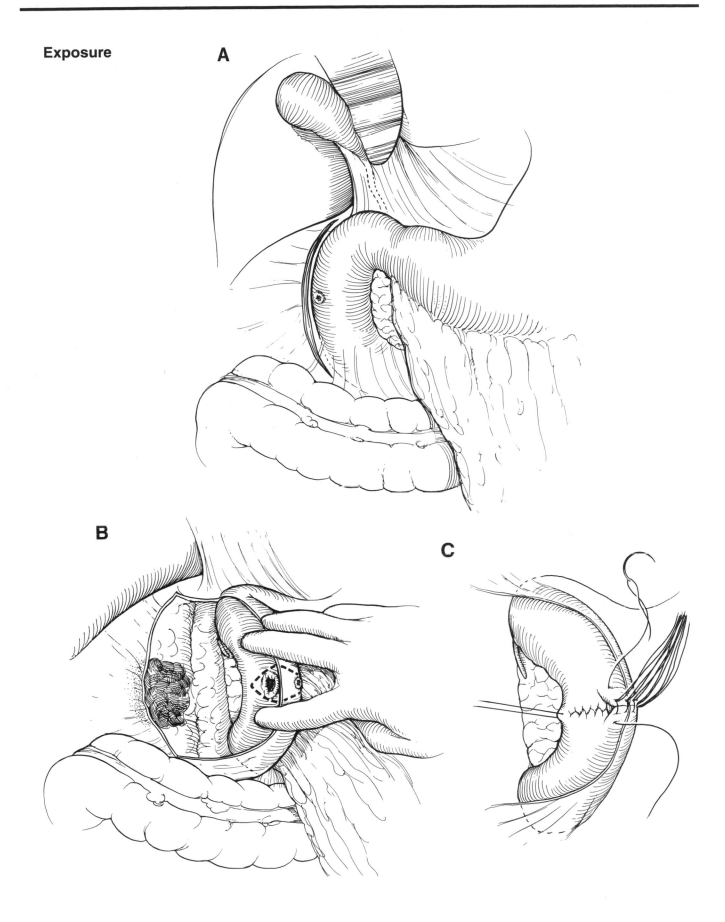

A

B

C

D. The third or transverse portion of the duodenum can be exposed by **(a)** removing the omental attachments to the colon, **(b),** taking down the hepatic flexure and mobilizing the distal ascending colon, **(c),** and taking the proximal transverse colon downward to the left. Care should be taken in the maneuver so as to protect the middle colic vessels in the transverse mesocolon. The peritoneal attachments of the transverse colon to the duodenum, if present, can be divided and the gastrocolic ligament divided if necessary. It is usually possible to take the gastrocolic ligament and omentum off the anterior surface of the transverse colon.

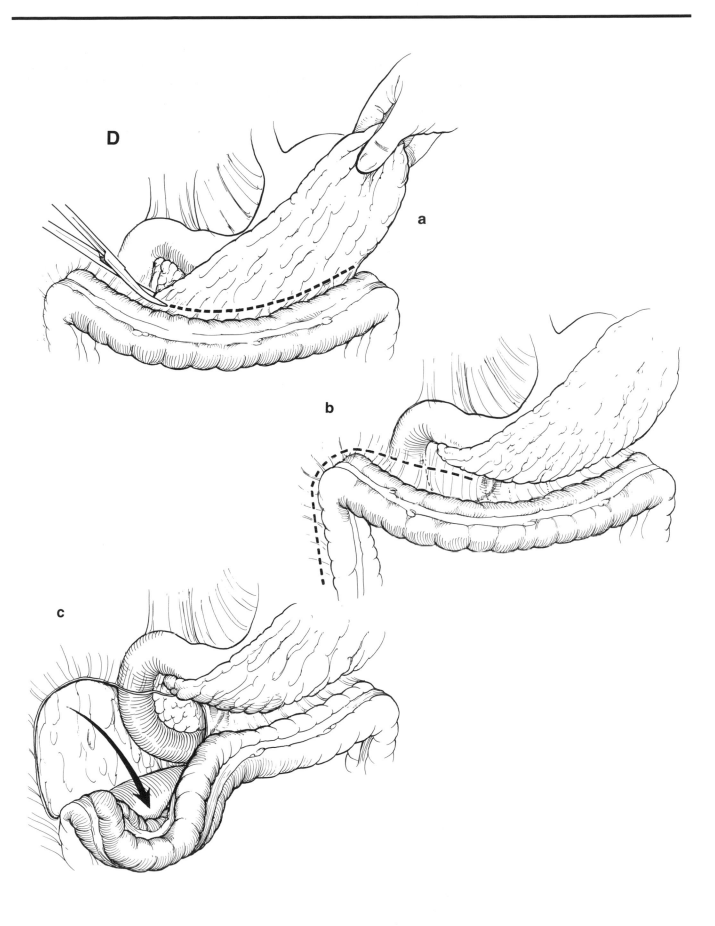

D

a

b

c

E. The distal part of the third portion of the duodenum and the fourth part of the duodenum and duodenojejunal flexure can be exposed by **(a)** taking down the splenic flexure **(b)** and reflecting the distal transverse colon and the proximal descending colon downward. The peritoneal fold attaching the colon to the spleen, the so called splenocolic ligament, should be divided, as should the gastrocolic ligament. This is usually best accomplished by taking off the gastrocolic ligament and the omentum as they attach to the anterior transverse colon. Again, care should be taken to avoid injury to the middle colic vessels and to the inferior mesenteric vein.

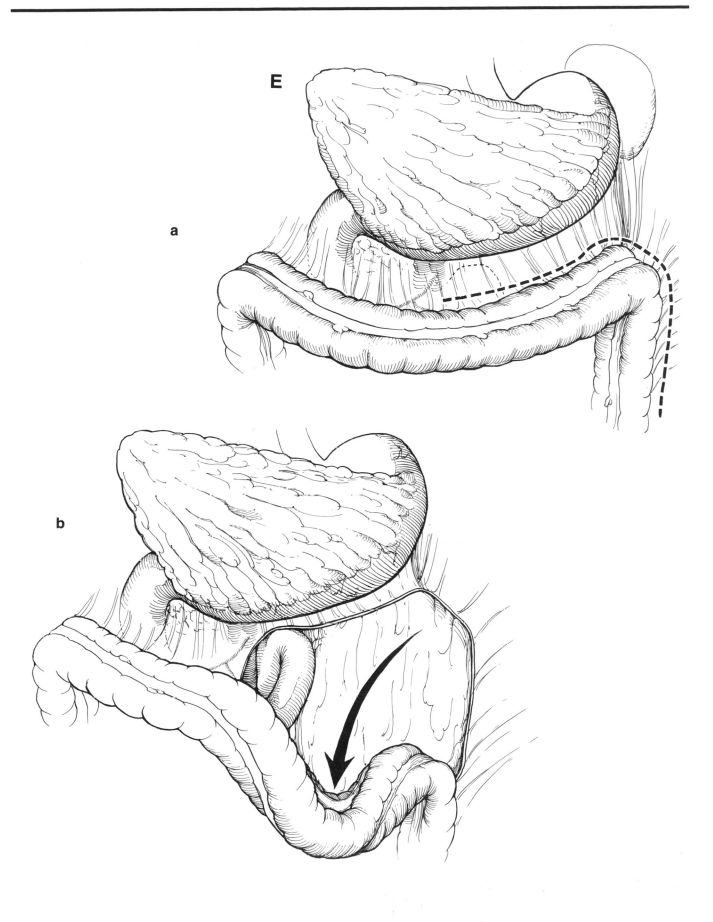

FIG 31–2

Duodenal Diverticulization

A. The technique of isolating the area of injured duodenum from the enteric stream (so called diverticulization) has allowed successful repair of some devastating injuries. This figure shows a primary suture repair of a combined blunt injury to the duodenum and pancreas resulting in a rupture of the descending duodenum and a hematoma of the head of the pancreas. The duodenal tear is closed with a running Connell suture reinforced by interrupted polyglactin sutures, but the closure is tenuous. The hematoma over the head of the pancreas should be explored with caution. If the pancreas is lacerated or fractured, great care should be taken to achieve hemostasis. When that is done, the surgeon should look carefully for ductal injury. A fine suture or two at the site of welling up of fluid is sometimes helpful. A Jackson-Pratt drain should be placed adjacent to the leak. All devitalized tissue should be debrided with meticulous conservatism.

B. Occasionally blunt or penetrating injuries may lacerate the pancreas as well as duodenum. Each of these injuries presents a highly specialized problem that must be handled individually. The principle is to avoid pancreaticoduodenectomy if possible, since long experience has shown the bad results of emergency Whipple operations. Do not be confused by occasional favorable reports of Whipple resections; the disasters rarely make print. Often a hematoma will obscure the extent of injury; in such case, the hematoma must be evacuated and the injured duodenum and pancreas carefully inspected. It is necessary to debride all devitalized tissue, but the debridement must be conducted with care so as to avoid excessive loss of tissue. We carefully debride to fresh bleeding tissue and then close the duodenum. Occasionally it may be necessary to ligate vessels between the duodenum and pancreas in order to get the duodenum closed. The security of the closure may vary and if there is any doubt, the closure may be buttressed by omentum or by a serosal patch, or the injured segment of the duodenum may be defunctionalized (all of these alternatives are shown in this section). The pancreatic injury should be appropriately handled by careful debridement and drainage as shown in **C.**

C. Every possible care should be taken to suture-ligate individual vessels and not just apply the electrocautery with broad strokes. When hemostasis is secure, careful search should be made for injury to the pancreatic ductal system, which is often revealed by the welling up of clear fluid. I rarely have been able to find the injured ducts. Even if I do find one and ligate it, I place a Jackson-Pratt drain adjacent to the pancreatic and duodenal injuries (as shown here) and bring the drain out a stab wound. If there is severe injury to the pancreas anywhere distal to the head, it may be advisable to do a distal pancreatectomy. We do not believe that it is a good plan to try to drain any distal segment of the pancreas into a Roux-en-Y limb. Leaks are common and the putative contributions of the preserved pancreatic tissue are not worth the risk.

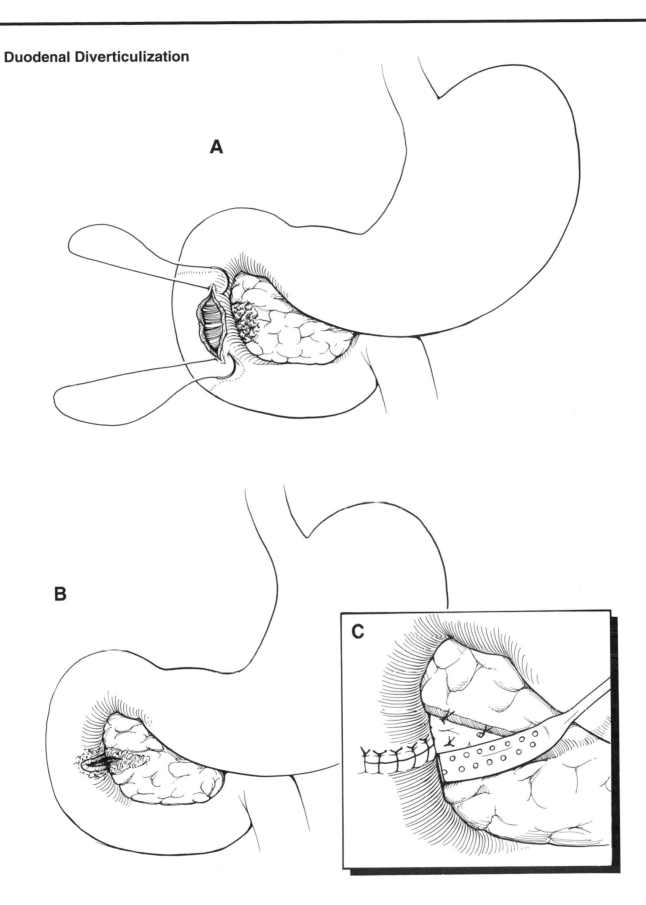

D. The actual diverticulization of the duodenum is accomplished by occluding the duodenum just distal to the pylorus and reestablishing enteric continuity by means of a gastrojejunostomy. This figure shows closing off the duodenum immediately distal to the pylorus with two rows of staples applied by means of the TA-55 apparatus. Another technique is to sew off the first part of the duodenum with a running suture placed inside the duodenal lumen via the gastrotomy wound created for the gastrojejunostomy. This can be accomplished with a running 3-0 suture that approximates the anterior and posterior walls of the duodenum just distal to the pylorus. Either way seems to work and common experience is that the proximal duodenum will reopen spontaneously months later (I don't understand this). After the duodenum is occluded, a routine antecolic gastrojejunostomy is accomplished by anastomosis of the stomach (just proximal to the pylorus) to a proximal limb of jejunum, brought up anterior to the colon.

E. Since the gastrojejunostomy is potentially ulcerogenic, we add a truncal vagotomy. We place a Jackson-Pratt drain adjacent to the duodenal closure.

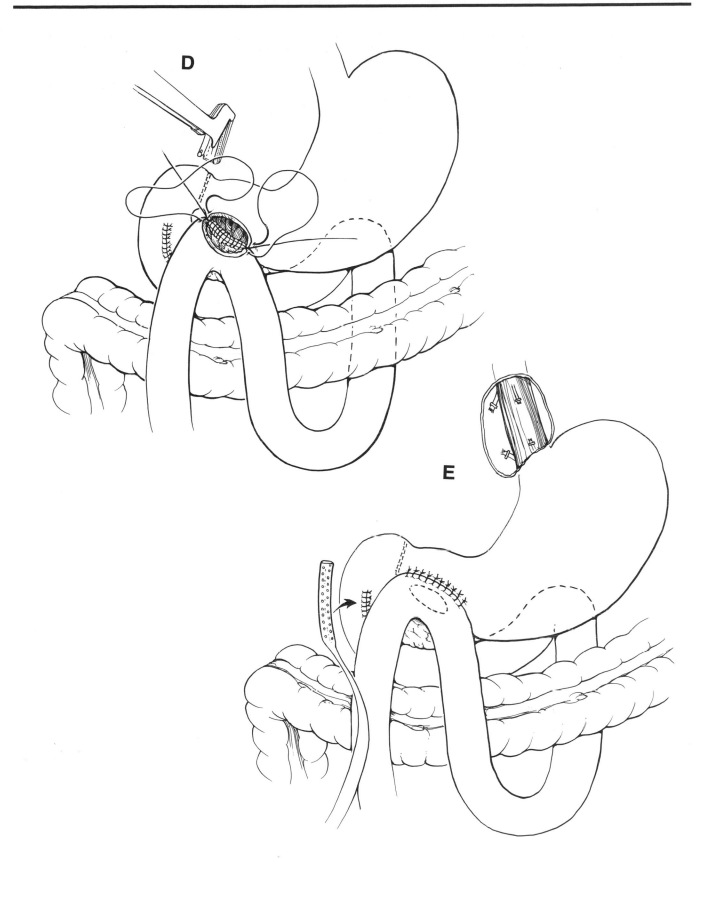

F. If the duodenal closure is particularly worrisome, a double-lumen Salem sump tube can be inserted into the proximal jejunum (see Witzel technique, **Fig 42–2**, p. 323) so as to allow aspiration of duodenal contents at a point near the area of injury.

G. Some surgeons have advocated a placement of a jejunostomy tube for enteric feeding distal to the gastroenterostomy. This figure shows the completed procedure, with the exception of the truncal vagotomy and the Jackson-Pratt suction drain tube.

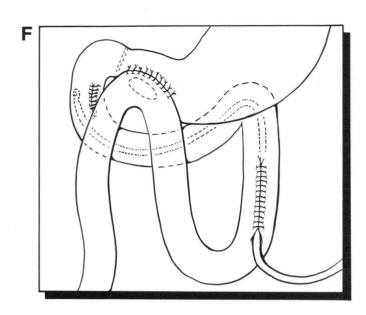

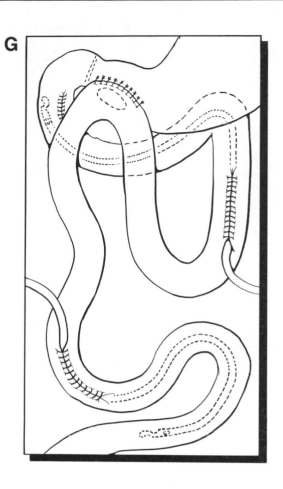

FIG 31–3

Repair by Roux-en-Y Duodenojejunostomy

A. One option with open duodenal wounds is to bring up a Roux-en-Y limb of jejunum and anastomose the open jejunum to the edges of the duodenal wound.

Repair by Roux-en-Y Duodenojejunostomy

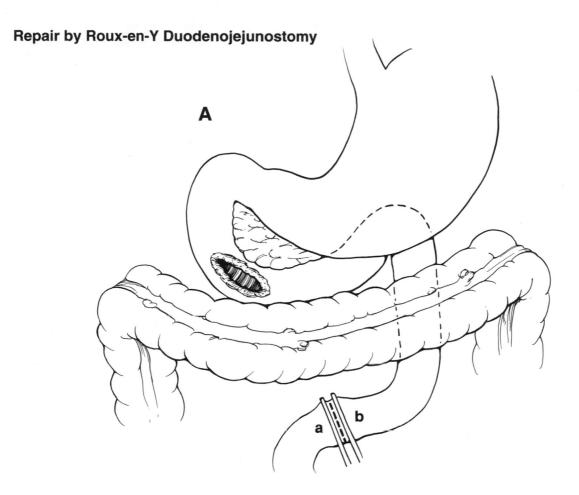

B. It may be necessary to tailor the jejunal orifice to fit the open duodenal wound. We use a routine two-layer anastomosis with a serosal row of interrupted polyglactin sutures and a running full-thickness stitch applied in a running locking fashion posteriorly, and then brought around anteriorly as a Connell suture. The anterior row is reinforced with an interrupted layer of 4-0 polyglactin sutures.

C. This shows the completed Roux-en-Y duodenojejunostomy. The advantage of this technique is that fresh tissue is brought into the area of the traumatized tissue for coverage, but the disadvantage is that there are two suture lines at risk for leakage. If there is question about the viability of the edges of the duodenum, or if there is an adjacent pancreatic wound, we often favor the serosal patch, shown in **Fig 31–4** (p. 233).

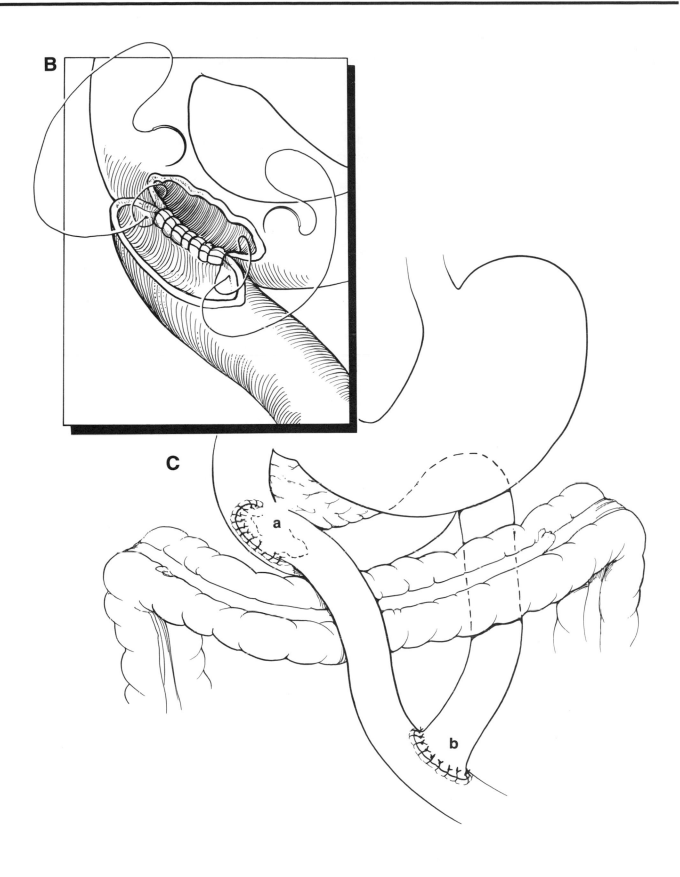

FIG 31–4

Serosal (Thal) Patch

A. Very large duodenal wounds often present problems in closure. One technique is to apply a serosal (Thal) patch.

B. In this instance, the jejunal limb has been approximated to the duodenum and rotated in a counterclockwise fashion so that it will remain untwisted when rotated here clockwise (bringing point *a* over to the medial wall of the duodenum adjacent to the pancreas). We use interrupted serosal sutures circumferentially applied in a fashion designed to avoid narrowing of the duodenal lumen.

C. This shows the closure of the duodenal defect with the serosal patch. Care should be taken to make the jejunal loop sufficiently long so as to avoid kinking.

D. The jejunal serosa closes the duodenal defect. Eventually, duodenal mucosa grows over the jejunal serosa. The method allows closure without great compromise of the duodenal lumen.

Serosal (Thal) Patch

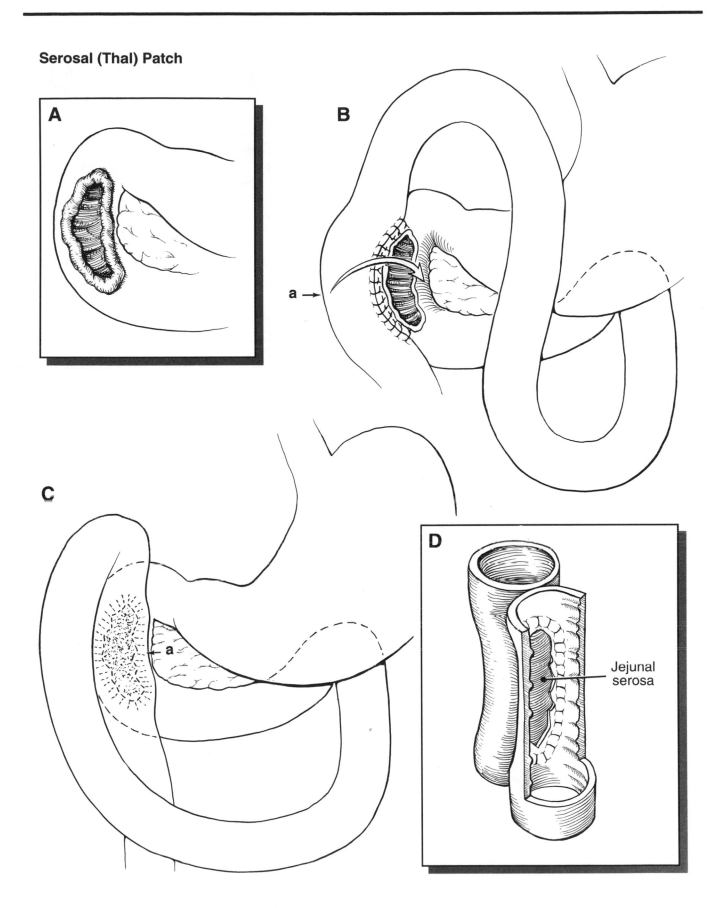

Jejunal serosa

FIG 31–5

Duodenal Hematoma

Blunt trauma to the upper abdomen may injure any viscùs by direct pressure. Occasionally, the descending duodenum may receive a blow that causes disruption of intramural blood vessels, resulting in a subserosal or intramuscular hematoma (shown here in frontal and cross-sectional views). If the patient is operated on for other indications, the injury is usually seen at laparotomy as a dusky swelling of the descending duodenum. Some controversy exists as to preferred treatment. Most believe, as I do, that these injuries do best if left alone; the hematoma will resorb spontaneously. The swelling is often great enough to block the duodenal lumen and some authors have suggested that if the patient is operated on for other causes, the hematoma should be evacuated, so as to rapidly restore duodenal patency. There is clearly room for judgment. If the serosa is split and about to break open, it may well be appropriate to evacuate the hematoma. At times, however, there is a tear in the mucosa and evacuation of the hematoma may lead to a full-thickness opening into the duodenal lumen, which may be difficult to repair because of the attenuated condition of the duodenal wall. All in all, it is probably best to leave the hematoma alone and allow for resorption. Enteric feeding may be facilitated by endoscopic passage of a feeding tube past the point of obstruction.

Duodenal Hematoma

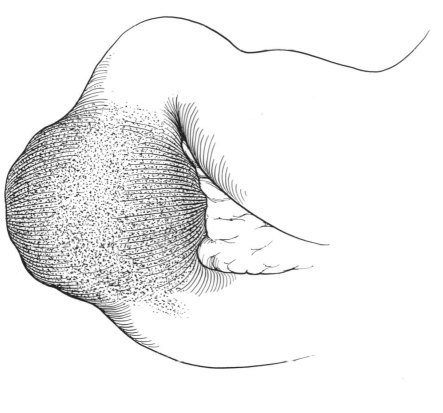

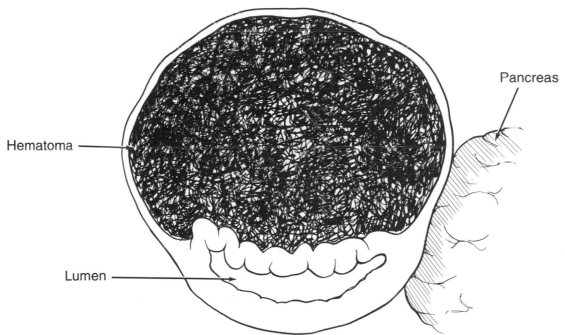

Pancreas

Hematoma

Lumen

Duodenal Polyp

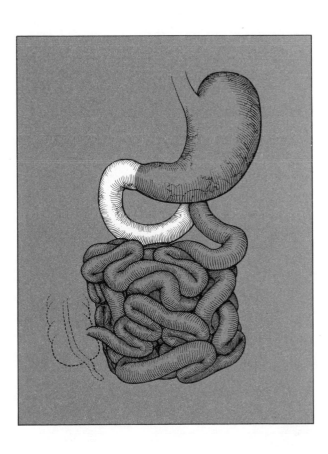

32

It is rare for duodenal polyps to be sufficiently large to cause any symptoms. If symptomatic, they may be removed by endoscopic snare, or they may be sufficiently large so as to be difficult to retrieve through the pylorus. In such cases, particularly if malignancy is suspected, they may best be removed at operation. As a rule, the question of malignancy can be settled by endoscopic biopsy; usually the polyp can be removed endoscopically. If not, we will operate.

FIG 32–1

A.   The polyp can often be palpated through the wall; it may be found to have a long stalk and actually to originate in the stomach.

B.   The duodenum is opened through a vertical (long axis) incision, the polyp is grasped, and a clamp is placed around its base. The polyp is excised and sent for a frozen section biopsy.

C.   If the polyp is malignant with stalk invasion, a Whipple procedure (Chapter 33, pp. 243–255) may be indicated. If the polyp is benign, the base is oversewn by placing a basting suture through and through behind the clamp.

D.   The clamp is removed and the suture carried back as a running locking stitch.

E.   The incision may be closed vertically, but if there is a problem with lumen size, it may be closed transversely so as to preserve the lumen. We use running swaged sutures applied in the Connell fashion.

F.   The closure is reinforced with a row of interrupted sutures. A good lumen should result.

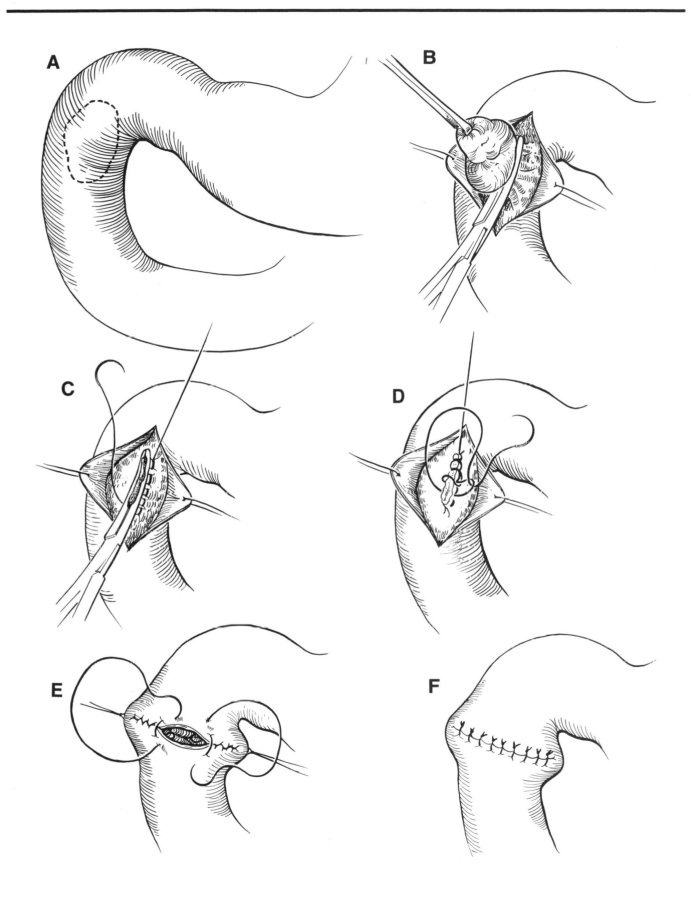

Radical Pancreaticoduodenectomy (Whipple Procedure) for Cancer of the Papilla of Vater (or of the Duodenum)

33

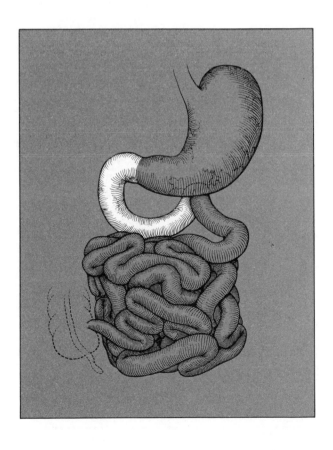

Malignant obstruction of the biliary and pancreatic ducts may be caused by carcinoma of the common bile duct, carcinoma of the duodenum, carcinoma of the papilla of Vater, or, far most commonly, by carcinoma of the head of the pancreas. All these tumors produce a well-recognized syndrome of obstructive jaundice, upper abdominal pain, weight loss, inanition, and often severe pruritus. The patient has acholic stools and bile in the urine. The term *Whipple resection* refers to excision of the head of the pancreas and duodenum and distal common bile duct. Total pancreatectomy is also used for treatment of carcinoma of the pancreas with varying frequency.

Here, discussion will be limited to malignant obstruction caused by carcinoma of the papilla of Vater or carcinoma of the adjacent duodenum, which are essentially indistinguishable in terms of the clinical syndrome produced. Of the four major causes of malignant obstruction of the bile and pancreatic ducts, patients with carcinoma of the ampulla of Vater have by far the best long-term outlook, followed by patients with carcinoma of the duodenum. Carcinoma of the distal common bile duct is a distant third and carcinoma of the head of the pancreas is, of course, the very worst of all. Differences in prognosis depend, of course, upon routes of spread of tumors, but also contributing is the salutory effect of the very early jaundice produced by tumors of the ampulla (salutory in the sense that the patient seeks help early).

Entire books are written upon variations in technique of Whipple resection. We will provide here a relatively straightforward technique for resection of the head of the pancreas, duodenum, and distal common bile duct. We will illustrate both the pylorus-sparing variant of the Whipple resection as well as the classic procedure of resection of the distal stomach with gastrojejunostomy. Similarly, we will illustrate three different methods for management of the pancreas: a side-to-side anastomosis between the pancreas and proximal jejunum, an opening of the pancreatic duct with an onlay Puestow-type of anastomosis, and exclusion of the exocrine pancreas by ligation or by stapling, without any anastomosis to the gut.

FIG 33–1

A. Carcinoma of the papilla of Vater causes early obstruction and dilatation of the common bile duct and pancreatic duct. Carcinoma of the duodenum gives rise to similar obstruction. Duodenal carcinoma may also produce symptoms of obstruction of the duodenal lumen itself. It is vital to determine whether a given tumor is capable of resection for cure. This is often a major problem in dealing with patients who have carcinoma of the head of the pancreas. However, in the great majority of patients with ampullary carcinoma the lesion is resectable, since jaundice occurs early and the patient comes early to operation. Diagnosis of carcinoma of the ampulla of Vater or carcinoma of the duodenum is made almost universally by means of endoscopic visualization and direct biopsy of the tumor, so that exposure of the tumor at time of operation is unnecessary.

B. The first step is to mobilize the pancreas and duodenum. The generous Kocher maneuver mobilizes the descending duodenum. The attachments of the duodenum to the transverse colon similarly should be divided so as to free up the second and third part of the duodenum. The lesser omental bursa is probably best entered from the left, dividing all attachments to the transverse colon and then using traction on the greater omentum to lift up the stomach and expose the pancreas.

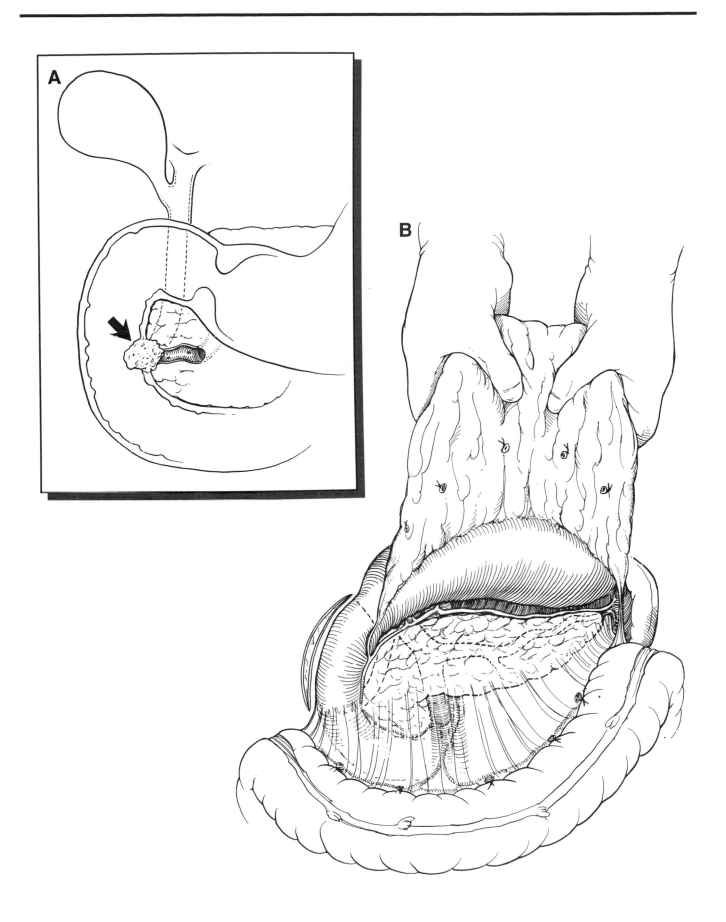

C. One of the classic requirements for determination of resectability is to exclude invasion of the portal vein. This freedom of portal involvement is usually easily demonstrated in patients with ampullary carcinoma and finger dissection from above just anterior to the portal vein and from below just anterior to the superior mesenteric will usually show that the tumor is nowhere near the portal vein. Many proponents of Whipple resection for carcinoma of the pancreas decry this step because of its difficulty, but it can usually be easily done in ampullary carcinoma.

D. Once a plane anterior to the portal vein and superior mesenteric vein has been established, it is possible to insert the small finger under the inferior surface of the neck of the pancreas and demonstrate clearly that the veins are not involved.

E. Crushing clamps are placed across the neck of the pancreas just anterior to the superior mesenteric-portal vein and the pancreas divided, taking care not to injure the underlying veins.

F. In my opinion, the most difficult part of the operation is freeing the posterior surface of the head of the pancreas from the underlying short, fat venous tributaries to the mesenteric and portal veins. These veins in the uncinate process and head of the pancreas are often wide, friable, and easily damaged. They should be approached with great care and all tears should be carefully and immediately repaired. Many surgeons prefer metal clips on the side of the superior mesenteric and portal veins so as to facilitate division of these short vessels.

G. This figure shows ligation of the pancreatic veins. Suture ligatures are often used on the side of the mesenteric or portal veins.

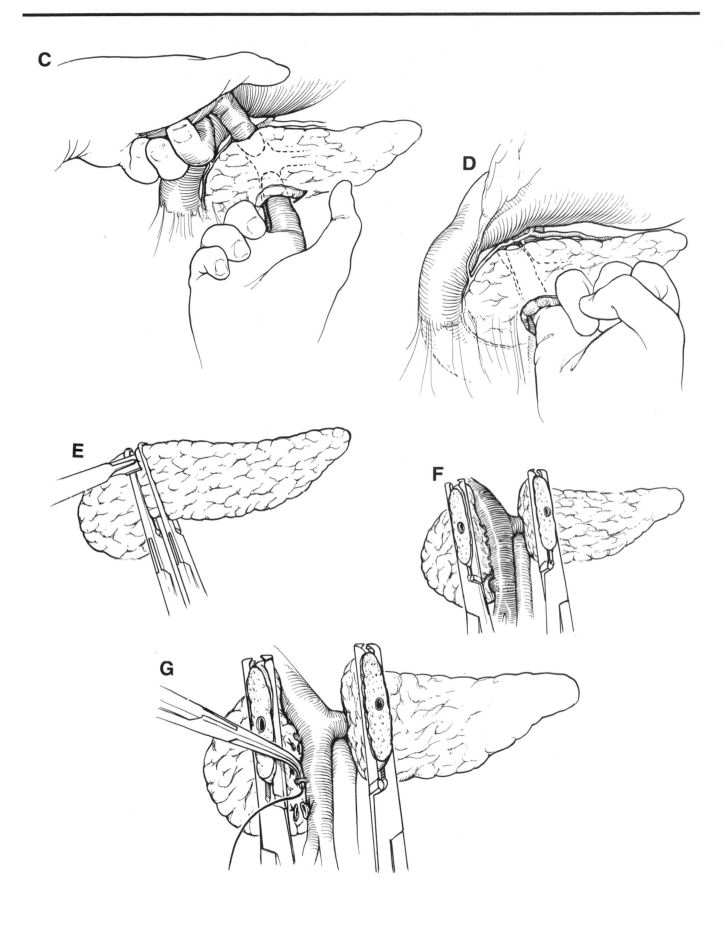

H.   This figure shows division of the dilated common bile duct just superior to the duodenum and transection of the gut about 2 cm distal to the pylorus. The pylorus-sparing procedure has been widely touted for its role in improving early gut function. I have not been particularly impressed by this change (we and others have noted delayed gastric emptying). I am not sure the procedure is superior. If we divide the distal stomach and take the pylorus out, we add a truncal vagotomy so as to mitigate against the chance of a marginal ulcer. Addition to this vagotomy may at times cause trouble with diarrhea, but diarrhea has not been frequent.

I.   This figure illustrates the alternative method of dividing the stomach at about the antrofundic junction. As you can see, the vagal trunks have been divided and a small Payr clamp is placed along the greater curvature just proximal to the proximal large Payr clamp. The stomach is divided along the dotted line and the lesser curvature side of the proximal stomach is closed after removal of the large Payr clamp. The small Payr will then serve as the anastomotic stoma for the ultimate gastrojejunostomy. After this step, the entire duodenum is mobilized around to the ligament of Treitz.

J.   A site is selected in the proximal jejunum about 5 cm centimeters distal to the ligament of Treitz and the jejunum divided with the GIA stapling device after a window has been created in the proximal mesojejunum. The duodenojejunal flexure is then circumferentially freed of and divided from all vascular attachments so as to facilitate delivery of the flexure and the immediate proximal jejunum into the lesser omental bursa by making an opening in the transverse mesocolon.

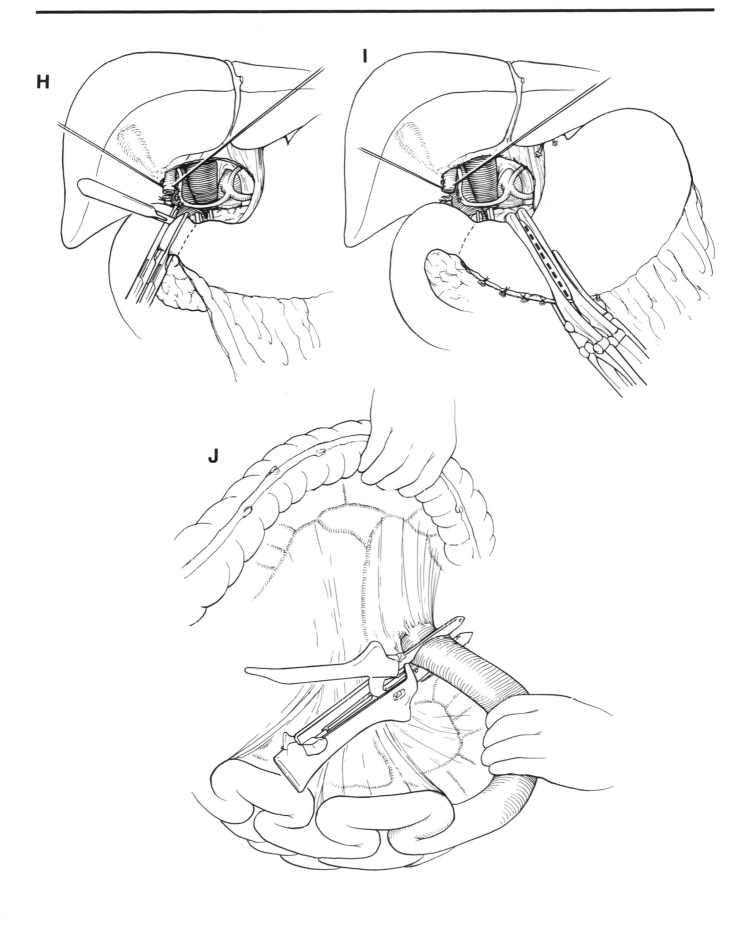

K. This figure shows removal of the operative specimen of the distal common bile duct, duodenum, and head of the pancreas in a pylorus-sparing operation. The proximal stapled jejunum is brought through the rent in the transverse mesocolon so as to restore continuity of divided structures by means of a choledochojejunostomy, a pancreatic jejunostomy, and a duodenojejunostomy. The gallbladder is usually removed separately, as it has been here; the *shaded area* is the gallbladder fossa in the liver.

L. This figure shows removal of the specimen in an operation in which antrectomy and truncal vagotomy were performed. The specimen consists of the gastric antrum, the distal common bile duct (not shown), the head of the pancreas, and the duodenum. The proximal jejunum is brought up through the rent in the transverse mesocolon for restoration of continuity with a choledochojejunostomy, pancreaticojejunostomy and gastrojejunostomy.

M. We anastomose the common bile duct end-to-side to the proximal jejunum using a one-layer running suture. The duct is sufficiently dilated so as to facilitate the anastomosis and to provide a good lumen. We do not use a stent.

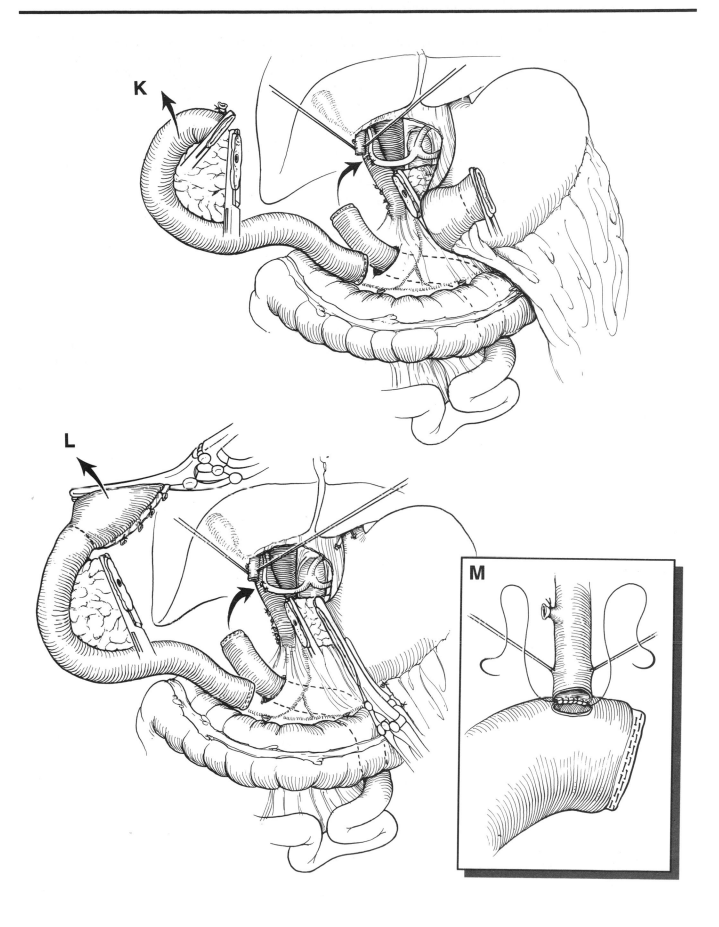

N. If the pancreatic duct is largely dilated, it may rarely be possible to perform a mucosal-tomucosal anastomosis between the pancreatic duct and the side of the jejunum. I do not favor this anastomosis, although it is used by many surgeons. The end-to-side pancreaticojejunostomy has a bad habit of leaking, which is often catastrophic. (If it does not leak, it often later undergoes stenosis.) The pancreatic capsule is loosely approximated to the serosa of the jejunum posteriorly as the initial step. After the end-to-side anastomosis of the duct to the jejunal lumen, the interrupted layer of sutures is carried around anteriorly, sewing the pancreatic capsule to the jejunal serosa, anterior to the ductal anastomosis. A common means of connecting the pancreatic remnant and the jejunum is to sew the end of the pancreas into the open end of the jejunum (not shown). Sutures hold so poorly in the so-called capsule of the pancreas that leaks are common.

O. This figure illustrates the completed so-called pylorus-sparing Whipple procedure with an end-to-side choledochojejunostomy, end-to-side pancreatojejunostomy, and end-to-side duodenojejunostomy. Not illustrated here are the Jackson-Pratt drains that we place adjacent to the anastomoses. The drains are brought out separate stab wounds.

P. This figure illustrates the completed Whipple procedure after antrectomy and truncal vagotomy. Shown are the end-to-side choledochojejunostomy, the side-to-side pancreaticojejunostomy (partially obscured here by the lesser curvature of the stomach), and the gastrojejunostomy, end-to-side, which we perform in two layers. Again, not shown are the Jackson-Pratt drains placed adjacent to the anastomoses and brought out separate stab wounds.

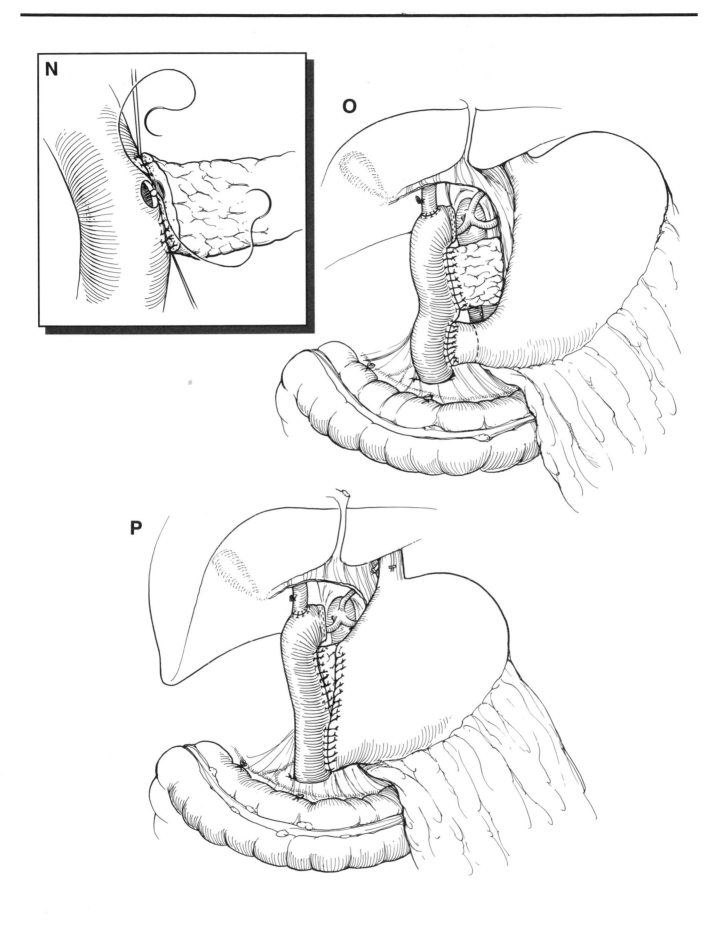

N

O

P

Q. An alternative method of creating an anastomosis between the pancreas and jejunum is to open up the distal pancreatic duct as illustrated, so as to create an opportunity for a side-to-side pancreaticojejunostomy, in a manner similar to the Puestow procedure.

R. In this side-to-side pancreaticojejunostomy, the posterior pancreatic capsule is attached to the jejunal serosa with interrupted sutures and the jejunal lumen is opened longitudinally so as to create a wide opening for anastomosis to the dilated pancreatic duct.

S. The posterior interrupted layer is continued so as to firmly attach the jejunal serosa to the pancreas.

T. The full-thickness anastomosis is performed in running fashion posteriorly with swaged 4-0 polyglactin sutures applied in a running locking fashion, and then brought on around anteriorly in a Connell suture.

U. The side-to-side pancreaticojejunostomy is then completed with anterior row of interrupted 3-0 polyglactin sutures. This is the anastomosis I now prefer. We then perform (in order) choledochojejunostomy and gastrojejunostomy.

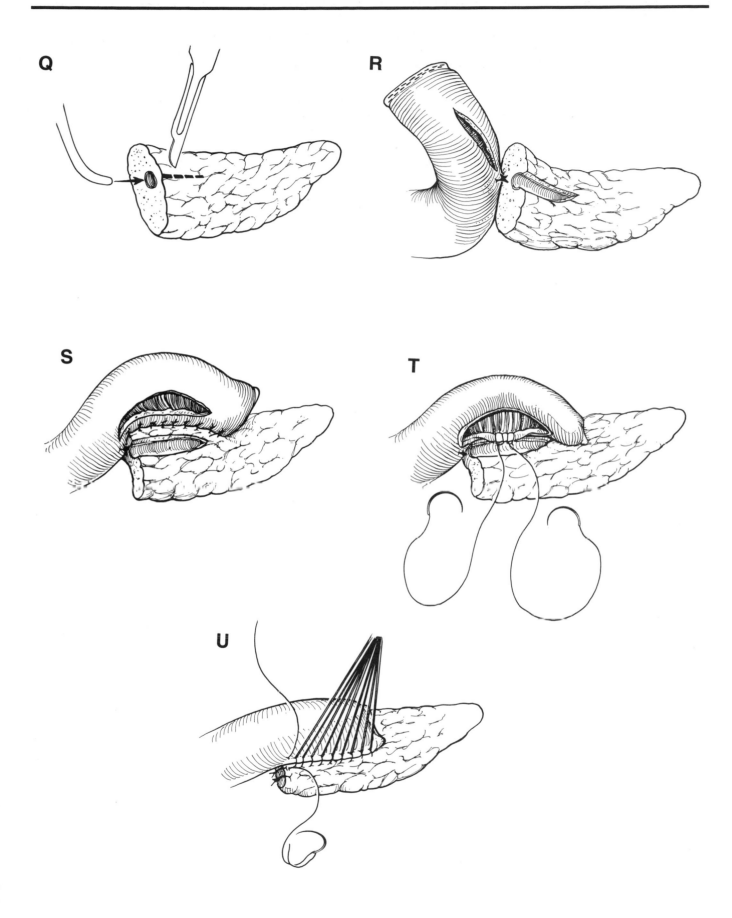

Q

R

S

T

U

V. This shows the completed Whipple procedure after vagotomy and antrectomy and the side-to-side pancreaticojejunostomy shown in **U.**

W. Some surgeons, cognizant of the late poor exocrine function of the pancreatic remnant after Whipple resection, simply ligate the end of the pancreas, and suture the dilated pancreatic duct, accepting the pancreatic exocrine insufficiency in trade for the advantage of diminished risk of leak of an anastomosis between the pancreas and the jejunum. Since such leaking is one of the main causes of mortality after Whipple procedures, many believe that this trade-off is a good one.

X. A double ligature is usually used, the pancreatic duct is sutured (not shown), and a Jackson-Pratt drain is placed at the end of the ligated pancreas.

Y. If the remnant of the pancreas is not excessively thick, some surgeons have used the TA-55 stapling device, although this produces rupture of the parenchyma and crushes a great deal of tissue. I have not used this technique.

Z. This shows the completed Whipple operation using the pylorus-sparing technique in which continuity has been restored with an end-to-side choledochojejunostomy and an end-to-side duodenojejunostomy, with ligation of the pancreatic remnant and placement of a Jackson-Pratt drain.

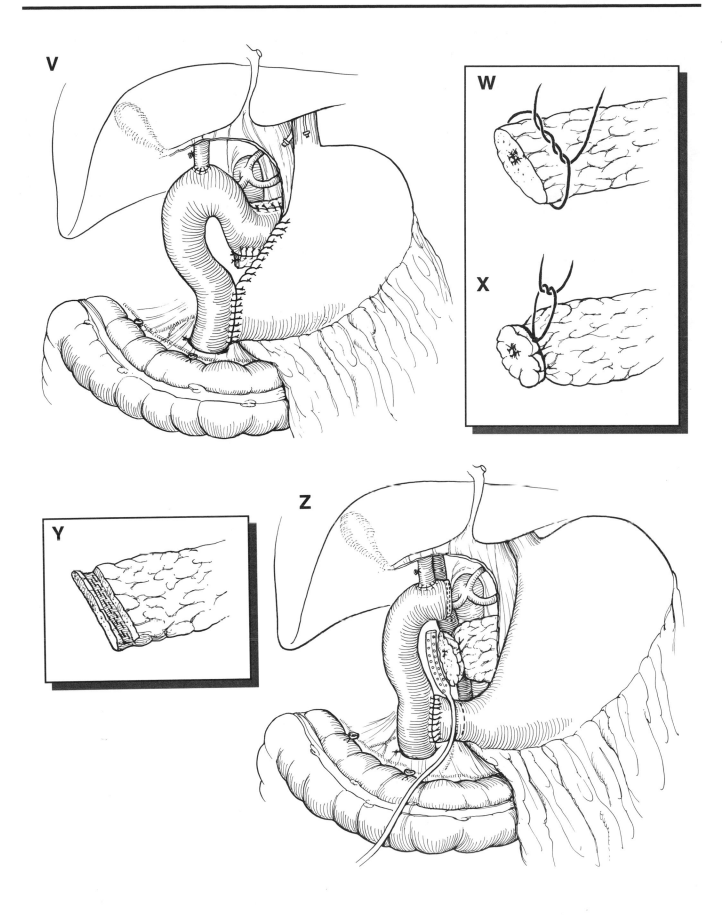

SMALL BOWEL

Mechanical obstruction is one of the most common indications for operation on the small bowel. Under mechanical obstruction we have included discussion only of adhesions, intussusception, and gallstone ileus. Other pathologic entities that may or may not cause bowel obstruction (hernias, tumors, and Crohn's disease) are discussed separately. At the end we have included a section on techniques in which we have arbitrarily included discussion of drainage of pancreatic pseudocysts—either cystogastrostomy or Roux-en-Y cystojejunostomy—since the topic did not easily fit anywhere.

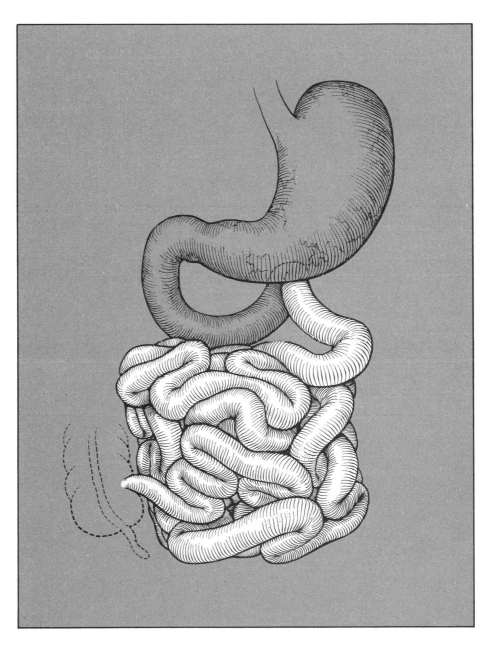

Anatomy
of the Jejunoileum

34

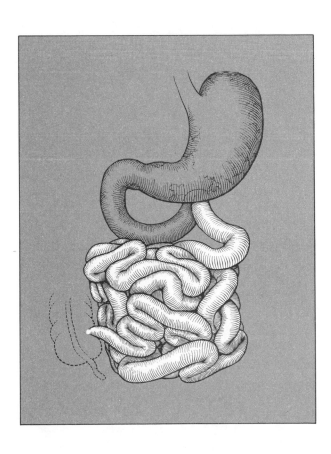

The only segment of the gut that is essential to life is the small bowel (footnoted disclaimers deal with intrinsic factor from parietal cells on the one hand, and with home total parenteral nutrition on the other). Digestion of food is achieved in the lumen of the small bowel and food is absorbed through its mucosa. In addition to its vital function in nutrition, the small bowel has other important roles. Among these: it is the largest endocrine organ in the body; it provides a vital barrier against infection and may be the most important organ in immune defense. It is a marvel of efficiency (failure of absorption of only 7% of ingested fat is regarded as malabsorption). The small bowel functions so well that, excepting the proximal 3 cm of the duodenum, it is not a common site for serious disease. We are supplied with a great excess of small bowel and can exist on far less than one half of the absorptive surface provided.

The truly impressive aspect of the small bowel is its immense mucosal surface area. Several layers of muscle, working with actin and myosin components in its microstructure, provide constant motility, so that not only is there great surface area, but the microinterface between the surface of the mucosa and luminal contents, presented for absorption, is in constant motion, facilitating contact.

FIG 34–1

A. The jejunum occupies the upper abdomen, particularly on the left side of the abdomen, and it is in contact with the pancreas, spleen, colon, left kidney and adrenals. The ileum occupies the lower abdomen, particularly on the right in the pelvis. It is relatively more mobile than the jejunum. The small intestine extends from the pylorus to the cecum. The anatomy of the duodenum has been described, and discussion here will deal with the jejunum and ileum. The length of the small intestine depends upon the state of bowel activity when measurements are conducted. The jejunoileum extends from the peritoneal fold (the ligament of Treitz) that supports the junction of the duodenum and the jejunum, downward to the ileocecal valve. Common estimates of jejunal length in normal adults are from 100 to 110 cm, and ileal length of 150 to 160 cm. The jejunoileum is estimated to make up about 60% of the entire length of the gut and to be about 1.6 times body height, so that the small bowel is considerably longer in a 7-ft-tall basketball player than it is in a 5-ft-tall jockey.

A

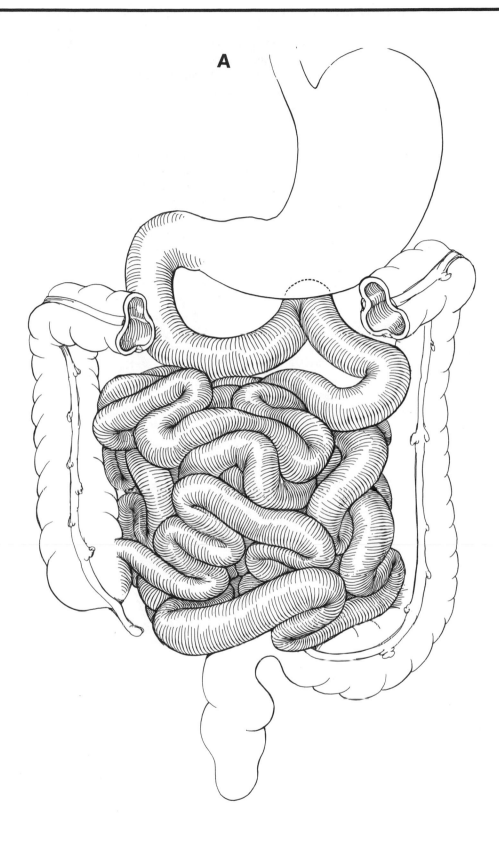

B. The jejunum has a larger circumference and is thicker than the ileum. It may be identified at operation because of this and because the mesenteric vessels usually form only one or two arcades and send out long vasa recta to the mesenteric borders of the bowel. Similarly, the mesojejunum is usually transparent, especially in the area adjacent to the bowel. Mesenteric fat may reach all the way to the bowel in extraordinarily obese individuals, but this is rare. The jejunal mucosa is relatively thick and has prominent plicae circulares.

C. The ileum is smaller in circumference and has thinner walls, multiple vascular arcades with short vasa recta, and abundant mesenteric fat that usually goes to the mesenteric border of the ileum. The mucosa is thinner and has few plicae.

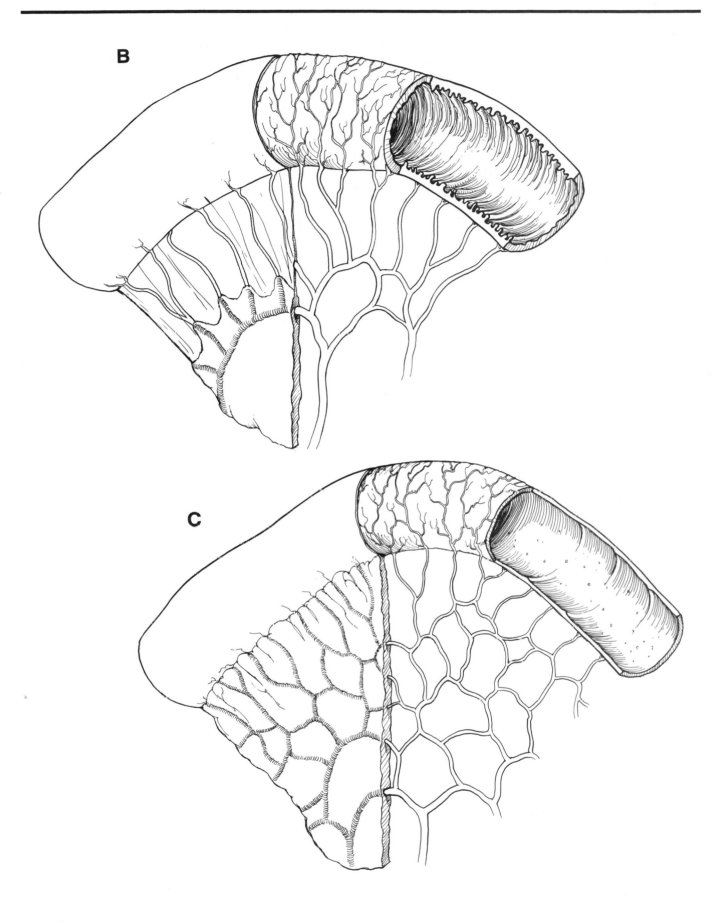

D. The blood supply of the jejunoileum comes entirely from the superior mesenteric artery, which also supplies the distal duodenum, the appendix, the cecum, and descending and proximal transverse colon. There is abundant collateral blood supply to the small bowel as a result of the vascular arcades in the mesentery, but in spite of this, occlusion of a major branch of the superior mesenteric artery, or of the superior mesenteric artery itself, will usually lead to death of the bowel. Venous drainage of segments of the small bowel is in parallel with the arterial supply; the superior mesenteric vein joins the splenic vein behind the neck of the pancreas to form the portal vein. The relatively high oxygen content of blood leaving the gut provides a significant proportion of oxygen supplied to the liver. If the mesentery is not greatly infiltrated by fat and if there are no adhesions, the bowel is extraordinarily mobile on its vascular tether, and in many individuals, jejunal segments can be mobilized sufficiently so as to allow anastomosis in the neck to replace the cervical esophagus. The small bowel contains major deposits of lymphatic tissue, especially in the Peyer's patches of the ileum. The rich lymphatic drainage of the small bowel plays a major role in fat absorption. Lymphatic drainage proceeds from the mucosa through the wall of the bowel to a set of lymph nodes adjacent to the bowel in the mesentery, from there to larger mesenteric lymphatics, to the retroperitoneal cisterna chyli, and from there to the thoracic duct. The lymphatics of the gut play a major role in immune defense as well as in the spread of cells arising from gut neoplasms.

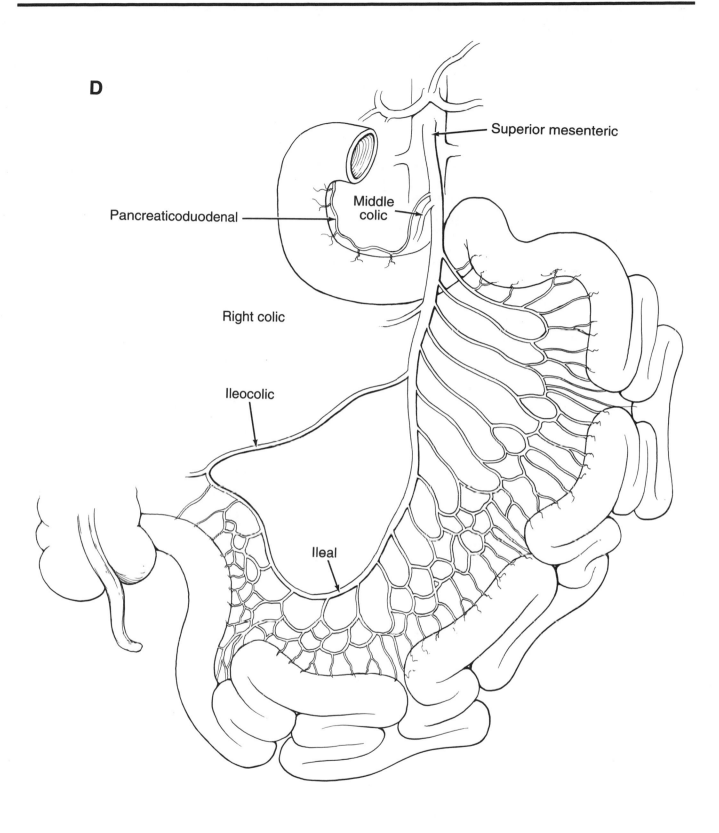

D

Superior mesenteric

Pancreaticoduodenal

Middle colic

Right colic

Ileocolic

Ileal

Meckel's Diverticulum

35

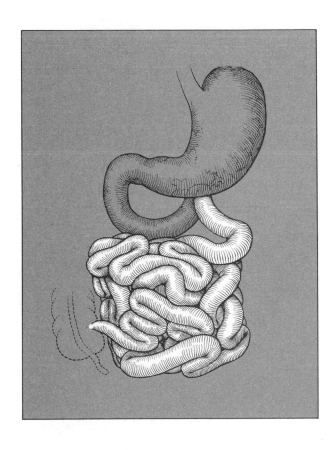

Meckel's diverticula are unusual anomalies arising from partial persistence of the omphalomesenteric (vitelline) duct. The usual manifestation is as a relatively wide projection arising from the antimesenteric side of the ileum, usually 18 to 24 inches proximal to the ileocecal valve. Occasionally, the diverticulum may be merely a small bump or hillock, or it may be long and narrow, but usually it is short and relatively wide. Various forms exist, depending upon the presence or absence of communication with the umbilicus or with various stages of atrophy of the omphalomesenteric ductal connection between the ileum and the umbilical skin (variations ranging from a persistent fibrous cord to a patent fistula).

The vast majority of Meckel's diverticula are entirely benign. Trouble arises from inflammation (which gives rise to a symptom complex usually indistinguishable from appendicitis) or from bleeding or perforation (usually caused by peptic ulcer caused by acid and pepsin secretion from ectopic gastric fundic mucosa) and from problems associated with persistence of part or all of the omphalomesenteric duct.

What should be done if a nonpathologic Meckel's diverticulum is discovered during laparotomy for some other reason? Opinion has varied as to the justification for empiric excision, but nearly all authorities now agree that if the diverticulum appears innocent, it should be left alone. On the other hand, if there is a persistent connection with the anterior abdominal wall (either a fibrous band or a persistent duct), the connection should be excised.

In excising a pathologic diverticulum, it may be possible, especially in cases of Meckel's diverticulitis involving the apex, to put a clamp across the base and simply suture the opening. Far more often, a partial excision of about 1.5 to 2 cm of ileum on either side of the Meckel's diverticulum with a formal end-to-end ileostomy anastomosis is preferable.

FIG 35–1

A. This figure shows the most common nonpathologic appearance of a Meckel's diverticulum arising bluntly from the antimesenteric border of the distal ileum.

B. This shows a persistent fibrous band connecting the apex of the diverticulum with the anterior abdominal wall at the umbilicus. The band should be doubly ligated and divided.

C. Bleeding from a peptic ulcer in a Meckel's diverticulum. This is an uncommon cause of occult gastrointestinal hemorrhage (seen especially in children) and the bleeding site may be localized by means of a radioisotopic scan. Treatment is to excise the diverticulum along with a small margin of ileum on each side and to do an end-to-end anastomosis of the ileum.

D. Rare twisting and strangulation of the diverticulum. Again, treatment should be partial excision of the ileum, division of the fibrous band at the anterior abdominal wall, and removal of the entire Meckel's diverticulum and persistent fibrous band.

E. A completely patent omphalomesenteric duct leads to appearance of enteric contents at the umbilicus. This requires excision of the omphalomesenteric duct, either taking the ileal end off flush with the ileum and closing it, or dividing the ileum adjacently on each side and doing an ileoileostomy. In either case, the umbilical end should be clamped and sutured, and the duct excised.

F. Cystic dilatation of the middle portion of the omphalomesenteric duct with fibrous atrophy of the duct at both ends. The cyst may become inflamed and perforate. It can be removed by double ligation of the fibrous tract, division of the tract, and removal of the cyst.

G. A variant of a persistent attachment of the omphalomesenteric duct to the anterior abdominal wall with a persistent tract in the wall, itself opening on to the umbilicus. This should be treated by excising the Meckel's diverticulum and circumferentially excising the persistent duct through the abdominal wall, taking care to remove all mucosa, followed by closure of the ileum and closure of the abdominal wall.

H. Inflammation of Meckel's diverticulum with a tip perforation. This will give rise to an appendicitislike syndrome. It is best treated by local division of the ileum, being sure to carry the line of division beyond inflamed tissue, and an end-to-end ileoileostomy.

I. This figure shows the suture line after local Meckel's diverticulectomy. We usually put a running basting suture behind a clamp, then invert that suture line with a row of interrupted 4-0 polyglactin sutures.

J. This figure shows a completed ileoileal anastomosis after excision of 1 to 2 cm of ileum on each side of a Meckel's diverticulum and routine two-layer end-to-end ileoileostomy.

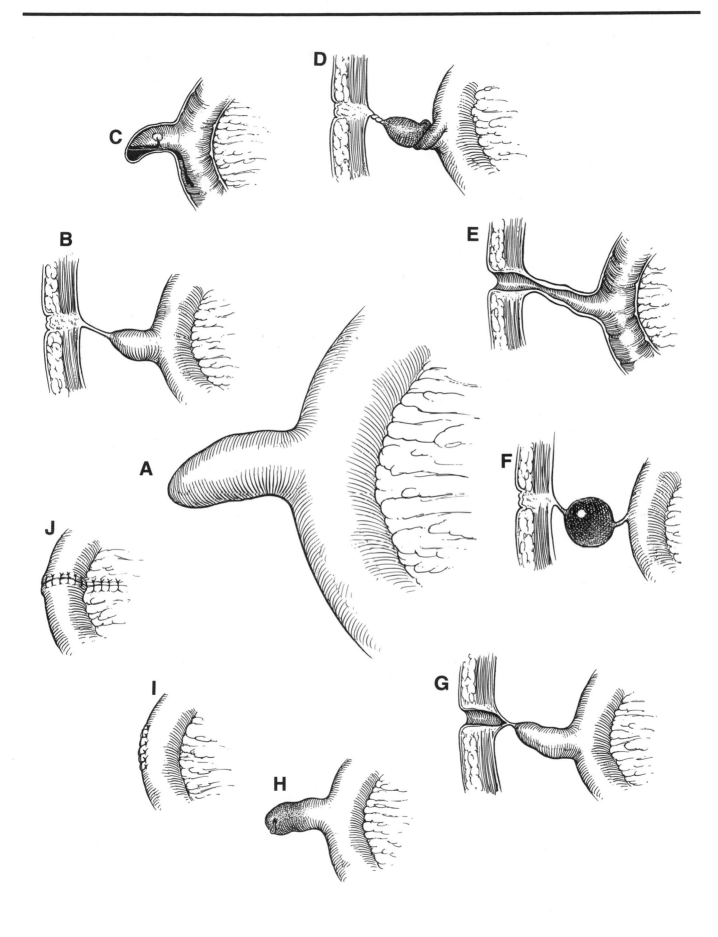

Management of Lesions at Ligament of Treitz

36

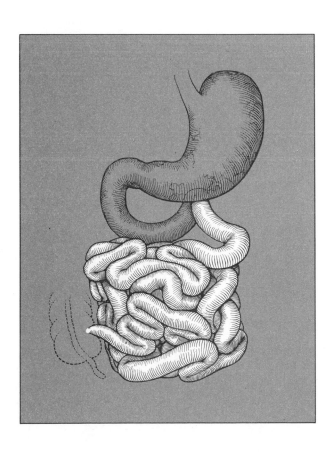

Tumor or trauma of the small bowel immediately adjacent to the ligament of Treitz often pose difficulties in exposure; resection is frequently difficult; and the anastomosis is hard to visualize, hard to accomplish, and apt to leak. A recent suggestion by Nauta (*Surg Gynecol Obstet* 1990; 170:172) may greatly facilitate management of these lesions and allow performance of a simple side-to-side duodenojejunostomy.

FIG 36–1

A. If the area of the duodenojejunal flexure is involved in a tumor, or angiodysplastic lesion, or trauma, or if it is adherent to a tumor of the stomach or colon or pancreas, or is subject to blunt traumatic blowout perforation, excision of the lesion (in the general area of the *star* in the figure) requires resection of the duodenojejunal flexure.

B. Such excision often leads to a difficult anastomosis that requires takedown of the splenic flexure of the colon, wide mobilization of the transverse mesocolon, careful dissection of the third part of the duodenum away from the pancreas, and an end-to-end anastomosis, in which the proximal end is usually fairly tightly tethered and difficult to mobilize.

C. Nauta's suggestion is that the offending segment be removed after division, proximally and distally, with a GIA stapling device, and with no attempt at end-to-end anastomosis. The divided third part of the duodenum is left in situ.

D. The proximal jejunum is brought up through the transverse mesocolon to lie along side the second part of the duodenum, where a large side-to-side anastomosis is performed. This does leave a blind loop of the third part of the duodenum, but the acidity of the contents of this area may inhibit overgrowth of bacteria. The blind loop should be kept in mind; if megaloblastic anemia develops, appropriate intestinal antibiotic therapy should be instituted.

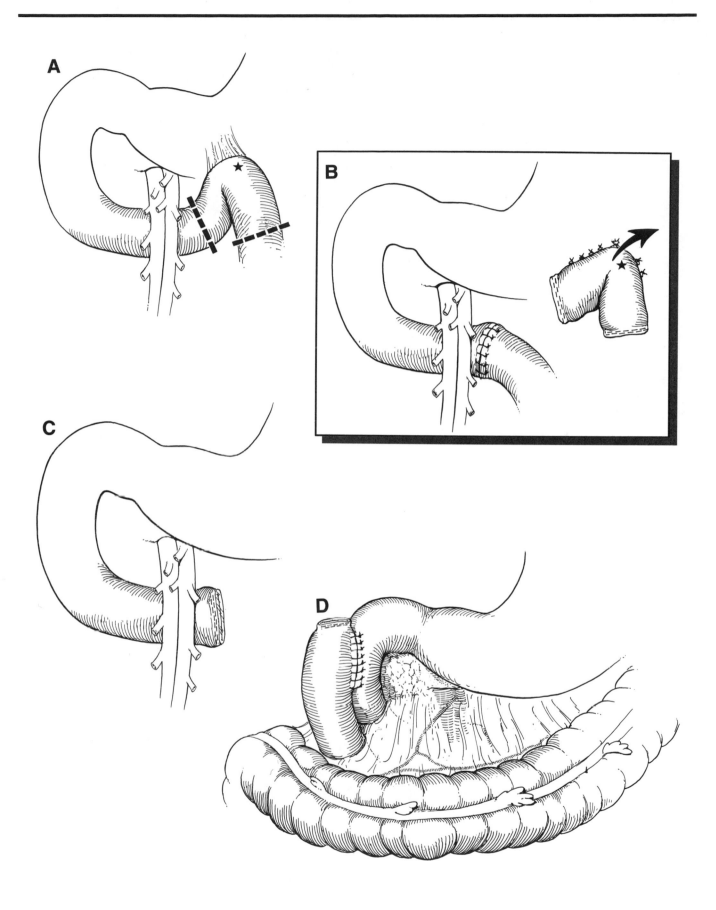

Small Bowel Trauma

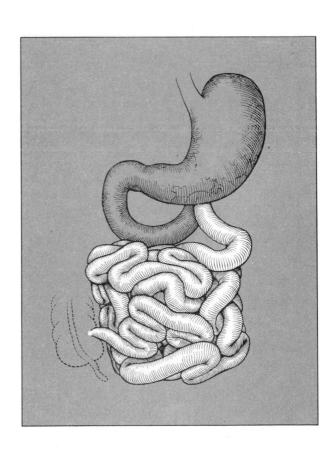

37

The small bowel may be injured by blunt or penetrating trauma. Since it is the largest organ in the celomic cavity, it is most often injured in penetrating trauma. The spleen and liver are more fragile and are therefore more often injured in blunt trauma, but recent surveys attest to the frequency with which the small bowel perforates after blunt trauma in automobile accidents. Perforation in blunt trauma may occur anywhere, but the most frequent site is about 10 to 15 cm distal to the ligament of Treitz along the antimesenteric border of the proximal jejunum. I don't understand the reason for this, but it is a true observation. In patients with crush injury of the lower abdomen, the mesentery of the distal ileum itself often tears as the bowel is pressed against the sacrum. Small bowel injuries after blunt abdominal trauma may involve only a small subserosal hematoma of the bowel wall or a small hematoma of the mesentery; often the trauma is sufficient to completely disrupt the small bowel. We have been surprised that there is often little enteric leakage in these instances, despite complete disruption of the jejunum. The bowel wall probably just goes into spasm. Repair of small bowel trauma depends upon extent of injury. Through-and-through gunshot wounds caused by low-velocity missiles may produce small, easily repaired enterotomies, but any wound with a missile of high muzzle velocity should be suspected of creating extensive tissue damage and the injured segment of the small bowel should be resected. In penetrating trauma it is important to carefully inspect the bowel for occult injury. Old-time trauma surgeons speak of the need to find an even number of holes in the small bowel, but occasionally a knife wound or a gunshot wound will tangentially perforate the bowel, causing only one wound. Multiple gunshot or shrapnel wounds will frequently damage many segments of bowel. The principles of therapy in such cases should be first to stop the bleeding, then to identify all perforations and areas of vascular compromise; next, all perforations should be temporarily closed with noncrushing clamps to minimize further contamination; next, decisions for treatment of each area of injury should be individualized. Here the principle is to close all perforations and excise devitalized bowel while preserving as much length as possible.

FIG 37–1

A. This is a typical blowout injury of the proximal jejunum caused by blunt abdominal trauma in an automobile accident. If the mesentery is uninjured and if the rest of the bowel wall appears absolutely normal, it is sometimes possible to repair this type of injury by local closure. In the vast majority of instances, however, the injury bespeaks tremendous local pressure. It is better to resect the segment and do an end-to-end anastomosis if there is any doubt.

B. This figure shows wounds of entrance and exit of a small-caliber gunshot missile. If the intervening bowel and mesentery are undamaged, we would close the two wounds locally.

C. In performing such closures, we would excise the margins and then close the wounds transversely, using a Connell suture of 4-0 polyglactin through all layers of the wall.

D. The Connell suture line would then be reinforced with a row of interrupted sutures.

E. This figure shows completed closure of the two wounds.

F. Large blast injuries are best treated by resection of the bowel. Often several areas are involved and require multiple resection. In such instances, it is of course important to try to preserve as much of the small bowel as possible.

G. This figure shows the completed repair of the injury shown in **F**.

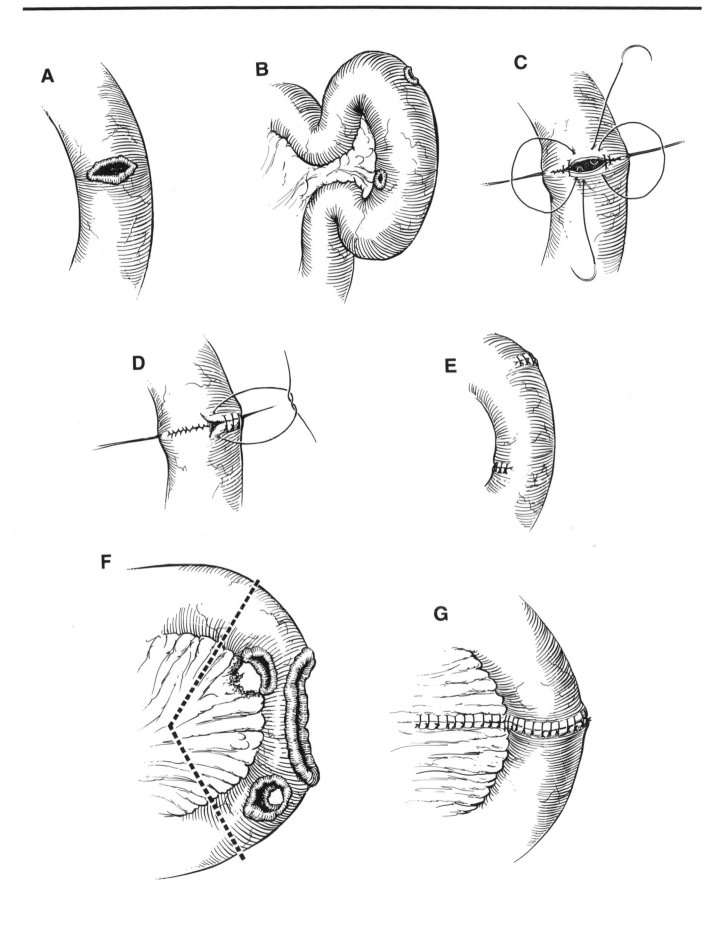

Small Bowel Obstruction

38

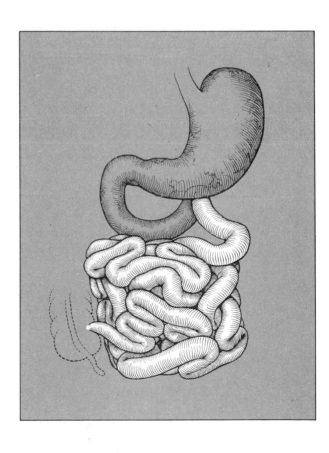

Postoperative Adhesions

Bowel obstruction may result from a wide variety of pathologic conditions. In North America and Western Europe, the most common cause of small bowel obstruction is postoperative adhesions, and the most common cause of large bowel obstruction is carcinoma of the colon. Adhesive band obstruction may occur without prior operation, rarely, in patients with prior peritonitis, especially pelvic inflammatory disease. Causes of bowel obstruction vary; in developing countries, phytobezoars are common causes of small bowel obstruction, and in India and Asiatic Russia, volvulus of the colon (sigmoid or cecal) is the most common. Years ago, Rodney Maingot suggested a useful mnemonic relating to the causes of bowel obstruction (both small and large bowel), which he called "The Rule of 12s." Briefly, he suggested that postoperative and other adhesions were responsible for 4/12 of bowel obstruction, hernias for 3/12, tumors for 2/12, volvulus and intussusception for 1/12, and miscellaneous causes (such as vascular accidents, foreign bodies, trauma) for 2/12. The flaw in this mnemonic is that, for example, tumors are common causes of large bowel obstruction and rare causes of small bowel obstruction; nonetheless it helps to remind us of the relative frequency of causes of bowel obstruction in our society. It must be successful, since I've remembered it for 35 years. We will consider intussusception and gallstone as causes of small bowel obstruction. Hernias, small bowel tumors, and Crohn's disease, which often cause bowel obstruction, will be presented separately. Obstruction to antegrade flow of enteric material initiates a series of symptoms that usually bring the patient to the doctor and may therefore be lifesaving. Since obstructed bowel often develops compromise of its blood supply (that is, it often becomes strangulated), symptoms that provoke early treatment serve a vital function. In Richter's hernia (Chapter 39), strangulation of the herniated knuckle of bowel often occurs without interruption of the enteric stream, and the patient may delay contact with a physician until after the knuckle is infarcted. Management of obstructed bowel depends on whether the bowel is infarcted. Sometimes infarction has clearly occurred, and we know to resect the dead bowel along with a short segment of normal tissue so as to afford good bowel for reanastomosis. At times, however, especially if the patient has been hypovolemic and if a general low-flow state has been in effect for some time, bowel ischemia is difficult to evaluate, and we cannot tell whether bowel is dead or alive. In such instances, we close the abdomen and plan for a second look in 12 or 24 hours, at which time the process has usually evolved to the point that we know clearly whether the bowel is dead or alive. This section deals with management of small bowel obstruction due to postoperative adhesions, with or without bowel infarction.

FIG 38–1

A. The small bowel is dilated proximal to the point of obstruction, in this case, a postoperative band adhesion. The distal bowel is collapsed. Occasionally, adhesions may be filmy and multiple, and it is often difficult to tell the exact point of obstruction since manipulation of the bowel may lyse the adhesions. In this illustration, the fibrous band is thick and tough and is divided by excision *(dotted lines),* whereon the distal bowel quickly enlarges.

B. The bowel underlying the adhesion should be carefully inspected, since there may be a zone of local ischemia that will give rise to later stenosis or obstruction, and it may be advisable to excise the segment. The bowel here is in good condition and needs no further treatment. It is important for the surgeon to examine the entire small bowel since there may be multiple adhesions and the obstructive effect of a distal adhesion may not be apparent.

C. Occasionally, a loop of bowel will herniate behind an adhesion and undergo obstruction, strangulation, and, as shown here, infarction. When that occurs, it is important to excise the entire loop of infarcted bowel along with a short segment of normal bowel on each side.

D. In performing an anastomosis between proximal obstructed bowel *(right)* and distal collapsed bowel left it is often necessary to spatulate the distal limb so as to provide lumens of similar size for anastomosis.

E. The completed anastomosis between the proximal dilated bowel and the distal collapsed bowel, which had undergone spatulation is shown. We do a routine two-layer anastomosis, with a posterior row of interrupted sutures and a mucosal-serosal row of running swaged sutures, applied posteriorly in the running-locking fashion, and anteriorly in the Connell fashion, then reinforcing the anterior row with a row of interrupted stitches.

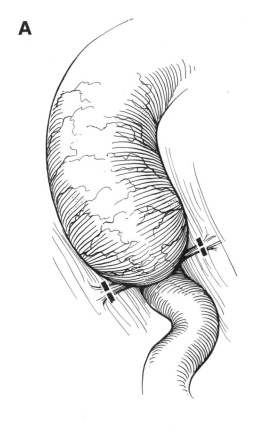

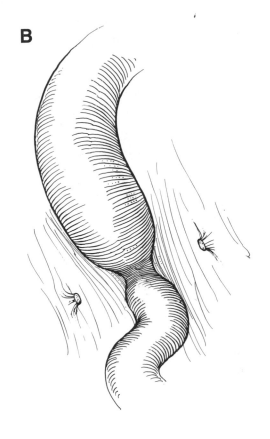

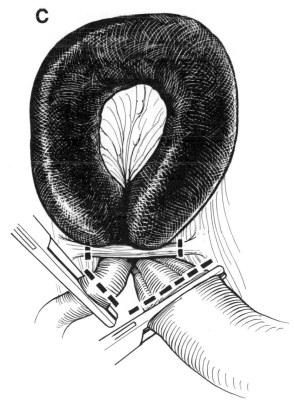

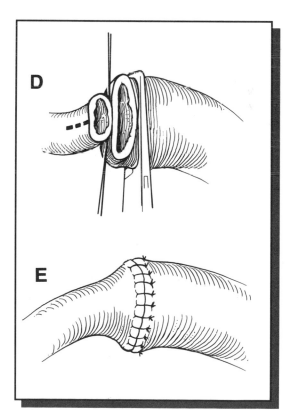

Intussusception

Intussusception is far more common in infancy (peak incidence, 3 months to 3 years of age), when it is almost always spontaneous, that is, the intussuscepting segment has no lead point. Various etiologic theories have been proposed, but none are yet accepted. Peyer's patches of lymphoid tissue in the ileum may serve as a lead point, but usually there is no detectable cause. Since the introduction of hydrostatic reduction (usually by barium enema) by Ravitch, the number and frequency of operations for infantile intussusception has greatly diminished. Nonetheless, in this country a large number of children are still operated upon because of failure to undergo successful hydrostatic reduction. The fear, of course, is that if the intussuscepting segment is resistent to reduction by increased intraluminal pressure, it may be strangulated or infarcted. The classic syndrome is the sudden onset of severe cramping pain in a healthy baby who may often pass clotted blood per rectum (currant-jelly stool). The symptoms are intermittent and often the child may go to sleep between attacks of pain. Barium enema is diagnostic and may well be therapeutic for the intussusception. In adults, intussusception is most always caused by some intraluminal tumor which presumably is caught by the peristaltic waves and moved along, dragging the attached bowel wall with it. Most all adults should be operated upon as soon as the diagnosis of bowel obstruction is made. In children, the most likely site of intussusception is ileocolic, although ileoileal and colocolic and ileo-ileocolic intussusceptions may occur. The frequency of intussusception in adults is low, and appears well-divided between small bowel and colon. Whenever intussusception is encountered at operation, gentle efforts should be made to reduce the intussuscepting segment by pressure on the distal bowel. Traction on the proximal bowel should be avoided. The amount of force applied should not be great and small amounts of pressure over several minutes is preferable to large amounts over a short time. Squeezing the distal segment gently with a sponge wrapped around the bowel may aid in reduction. If the intussusception fails to reduce, the segment should be excised. Since tumors are commonly involved in adult intussusception, we usually make a wider resection in adults. If, after manual reduction, the reduced segment appears to have its blood supply compromised, resection may still be necessary. If the segment is clearly infarcted it should be excised. If there is doubt, we usually put warm sponges on the bowel and wait a while. If doubt persists, one should go ahead with resection, although it is usually not necessary to resect bowel that will reduce.

FIG 38–2

A.   This figure illustrates a classic spontaneous ileocolic intussusception in an infant. The intussusception may well go all the way around to the transverse colon. On entering the abdomen, it may be possible to reduce the intussusception into the ascending colon by means of pressure on the leading point with two fingers inserted into the small abdominal wound. If necessary, the right colon can be mobilized and pressure applied with the thumb and forefingers of both hands against the leading point, so as to gently reduce the intussusception. Failure to reduce usually means that there is some serious problem and resection may be

B.   This figure illustrates an irreducible ileocolic intussusception treated by local excision of the terminal ileum and ascending colon. Continuity is restored with an ileocolostomy, usually one-layer fine silk suture.

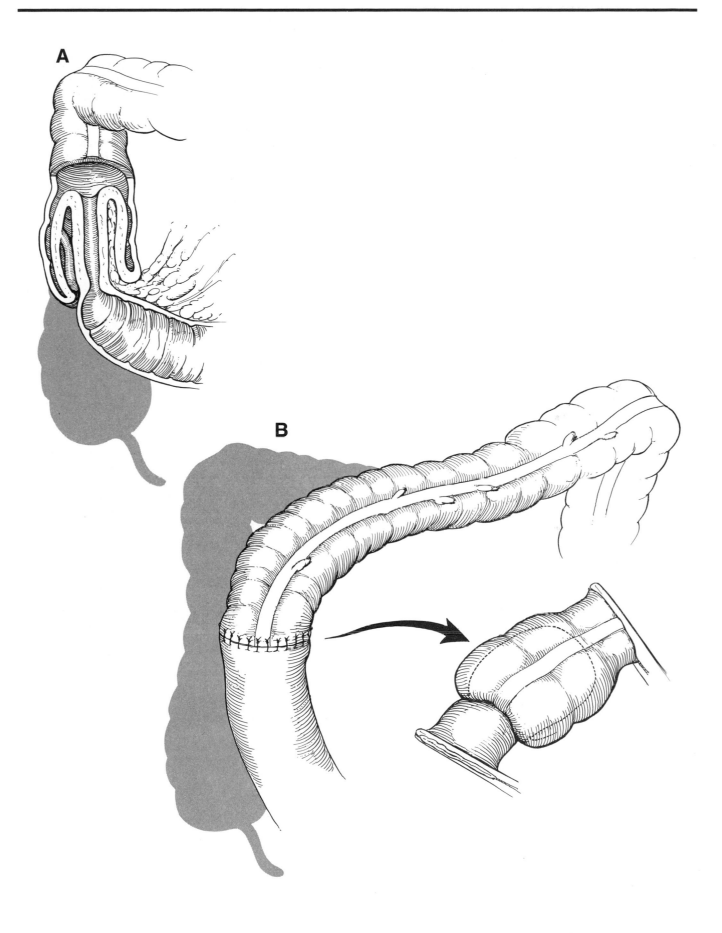

C. This figure illustrates an ileoileal intussusception with an ileal tumor as the lead point. The lesion is usually found in adults and it may be possible to reduce the intussuscepting segment. If the segment did reduce easily, we would then go ahead with a resection to remove the tumor, taking care to get adequate margins and a good wedge of mesentery. The obstructed proximal bowel is dilated and the distal bowel collapsed, so that it will be necessary to tailor the anastomosis in order to manage the discrepancy in size.

D. This is an ileocolic intussusception in an adult with a tumor at the lead point.

E. Again, attempts should be made by general pressure to reduce the intussusception.

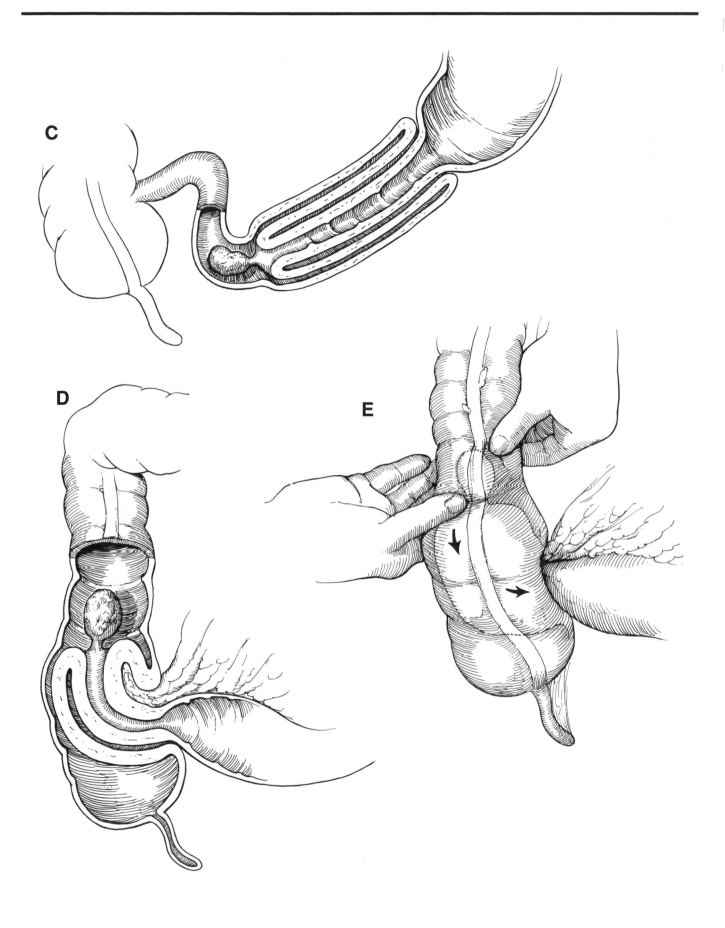

F. This shows a colocolic intussusception of a tumor from the hepatic flexure into the transverse colon in an adult. We would certainly make preliminary efforts at reduction, but unless the reduction were almost spontaneous, we would go ahead with a right colectomy and anastomose the terminal ileum to the left transverse colon.

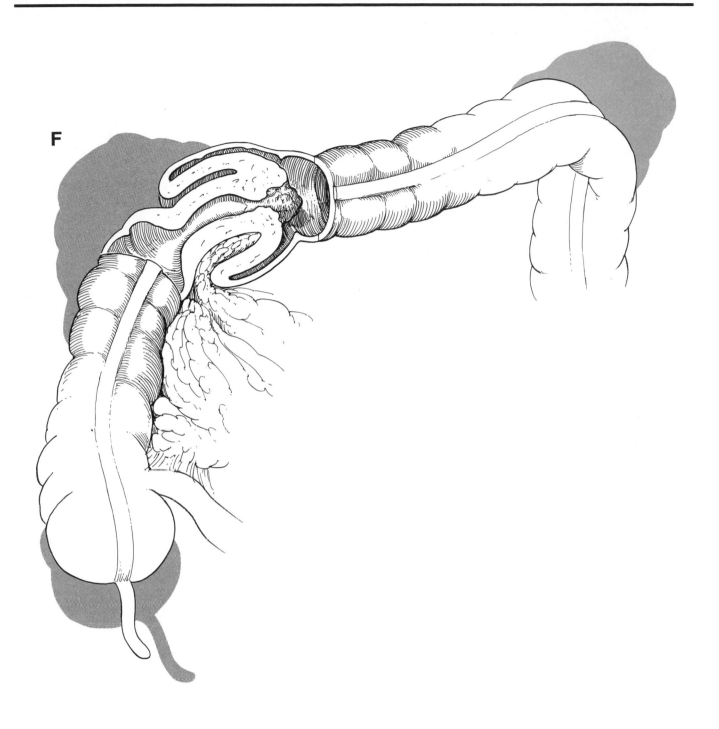

F

Gallstone Ileus

Gallstone ileus is a rare cause of bowel obstruction. Obstruction results, of course, from obturation of the distal small bowel by a gallstone that has passed from the gallbladder into the bowel via a cholecystoenteric (usually duodenal) fistula. The diagnosis can be made pre-operatively by determining that the patient does have small bowel obstruction, and occasionally, by seeing streaks of air within the liver (so-called air cholangiogram), as well as occasionally, by visualizing the gallstone itself. Although only 15% of gallstones are said to be radiopaque, by the time they achieve sufficient size so as to cause bowel obstruction, they usually contain enough calcium to be seen. The problem is that they often overlie the sacrum or sacroiliac junction, and may often be seen only on lateral x-ray views of the abdomen. The question that arises is: once the obstructing gallstone is removed, should the gallbladder be excised and the cholecystoenteric fistula repaired? The answer depends entirely upon the condition of the patient. The patient is often old, fragile, and in poor condition, in which case the surgeon's commission is to relieve the threat to life, that is, the bowel obstruction; fixing the cholecystoenteric fistula can wait until later. The recent trend, however, has been to do the whole procedure at once. Such an accomplishment is commendable if done without serious risk to the patient.

FIG 38–3

A. A cholecystoenteric fistula is usually the result of acute cholecystitis with localized gangrene, which causes adherence of the gallbladder to the bowel. Pressure necrosis of the tissue separating the gallbladder and bowel lumen causes the fistulous opening.

B. After the stone enters the duodenum, the fistulous opening between the gallbladder and duodenum persists. The gallstone is carried distally by peristalsis.

C. The gallstone often may traverse the entire gut and be passed via the anus. If the stone is large enough to cause obturator obstruction, the obstruction usually occurs 5 to 15 cm proximal to the ileocecal valve. The patient develops classic signs of small bowel obstruction with great abdominal distention and relatively late vomiting.

D. At operation for gallstone ileus, the gallstone should be located and gently milked in a retrograde fashion away from the spot of impaction. The exact area of impaction is often ulcerated and the bowel wall is thin. The stone should be passed retrograde to a point where the inflammation is not great and the edema is less pronounced. An enterotomy should be made at that site and the stone extracted.

E. After the gallstone is removed, the enterotomy should be closed in two layers. Careful search should be made throughout the bowel for a possible second stone (or multiple stones) before the enterotomy is closed. If the patient is doing well at this point, we take down the cholecystoduodenal fistula, perform a cholecystectomy, and close the opening into the duodenum. If this opening is large and fibrotic, we may buttress the closure with a serosal patch by bringing up a loop of jejunum and sewing the jejunal serosa around the duodenal closure (see Chapter 31 on duodenal trauma).

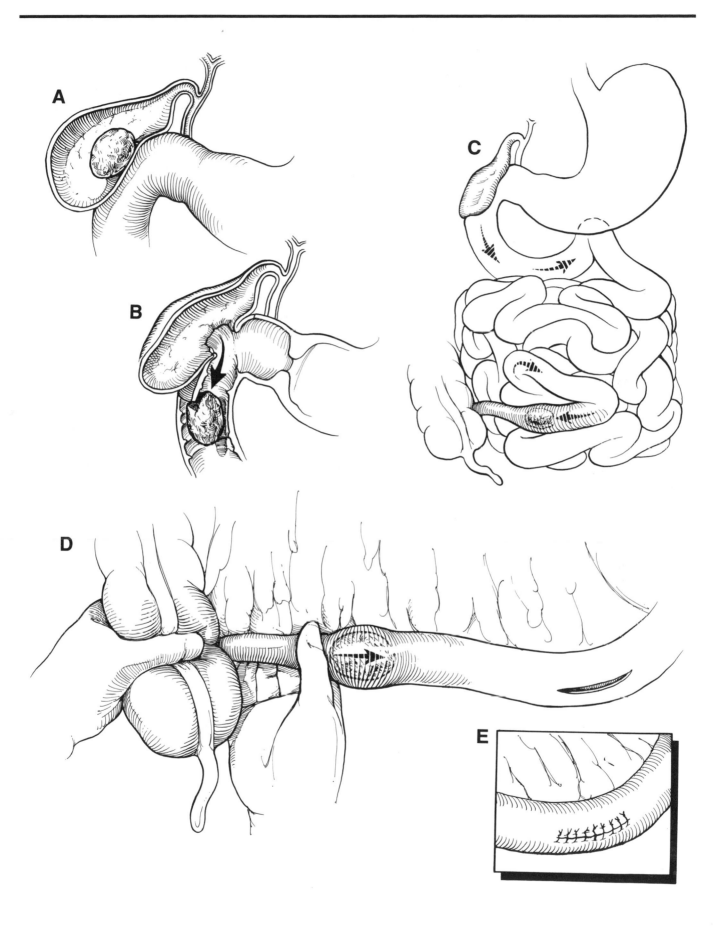

Small Bowel in Hernias: Indirect Inguinal, Richter's, and Femoral

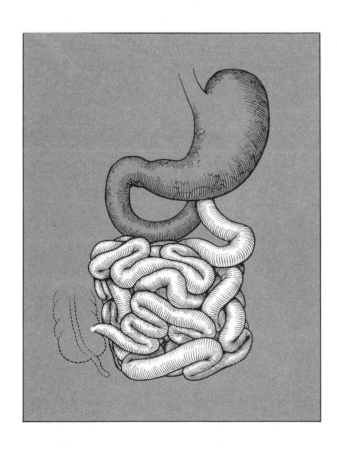

39

Discussions of diagnosis and repair of abdominal wall hernias are not within our present scope, but it is certainly clear that the most common serious complication of hernias in the abdominal wall is incarceration and strangulation of small bowel. I will briefly discuss hernias from the standpoint of risks to the small intestine. Presentation will be limited to common groin hernias.

FIG 39-1

A. The hernial sac in indirect inguinal hernias is developed from a persistent peritoneal processus vaginalis, a small tubular projection of the peritoneum that follows the migration of the testicle into the scrotum in intrauterine life; when the migration is complete, the processus is usually obliterated. The illustration shows a loop of mobile ileum protruding through the internal and external inguinal rings within the hernia sac down into the superior aspect of the scrotum. The bowel is contained in a peritoneal sac that is actually a persistent patent processus vaginalis.

B. If the blood supply to the segment of bowel trapped in the hernia is compromised by twisting or swelling, the venous and lymphatic drainage will be impeded and the volume of the bowel will increase greatly as more blood enters the loop than leaves it. Within a variable time, pressure within the bowel interstitium will so increase as to further compromise the venous limb of the Starling circulatory loop, leading to further increased pressure and hypoxia. The loop of bowel is said to be strangulated. If the process continues, the loop will die. Rescue can be provided by herniorrhaphy, that is, by opening the inguinal canal, reducing the hernia, reinserting the bowel into the abdominal cavity through the internal inguinal ring (provided, of course, that the bowel is viable), ligation of the hernia sac near the internal inguinal ring, and repairing the hernia defect by one of several methods (such as those of Bassini, Halsted, or Ferguson). Infarcted bowel should be excised and gut continuity reestablished. If viability is questionable, we perform a second look in 18 to 24 hours.

C. An unusual complication of abdominal wall hernias, seen especially in femoral hernias, is protrusion of a portion of the circumference of the wall of the bowel through the hernial defect (the so-called Richter's hernia). This condition is particularly dangerous. Ordinarily, compromise of the blood supply of the bowel is immediately followed by bowel obstruction, and the symptoms that ensue usually cause the patient quickly to seek help. Since only a portion of the bowel circumference is involved in a Richter's hernia, however, the enteric stream may be uninterrupted, even though the small knuckle of bowel may strangulate and undergo necrosis and ultimately perforate and cause death. Reduction may be difficult and a segment containing the strangulated Richter's hernia often requires resection, to be followed by a Cooper's ligament repair, if the original defect was a femoral hernia.

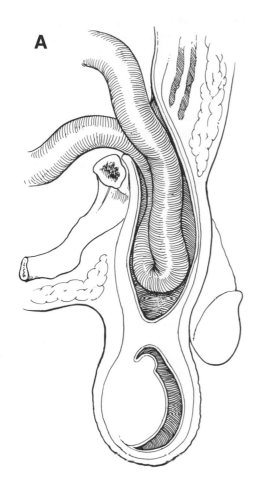

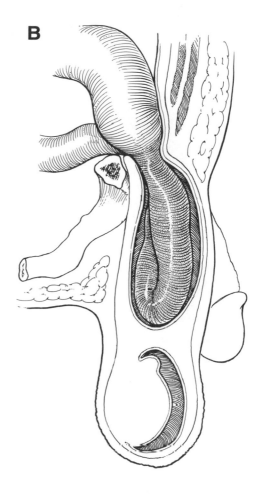

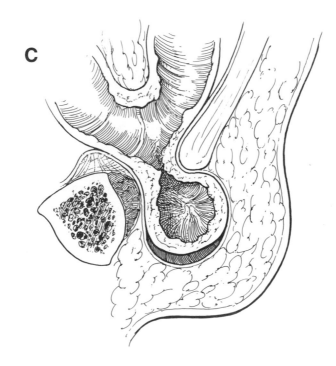

D. Figures **D** through **G** refer to femoral hernias. Hernias through the femoral canal are not nearly as common as inguinal hernias. Because of the rigidity of the abdominal wall outlet, the neck of the hernial sac is narrow, and if a loop of bowel protrudes through it, it is often subject to strangulation. Diagnosis of femoral hernias may be difficult, and at times they may be impossible to distinguish from enlarged, tender femoral lymph nodes.

E. The best operative approach is through an inguinal incision. This shows an opening in the external oblique aponeurosis, which is held up by forceps (tips shown). The conjoined tendon is shown curving above, and the instrument is placed through the transversalis fascia, inferior to the conjoined tendon, through the femoral canal under the inguinal ligament, to grasp the sac of the femoral hernia. If the sac is enlarged, this reduction may not be possible and division of the inguinal ligament may be necessary. Division should cause no concern.

F. Once the sac is reduced, it should be opened and the hernial contents inspected. If the contents show no evidence of vascular insufficiency, they should be replaced within the peritoneal cavity.

G. The hernial sac, once emptied, should be twisted and transfixed at its base and severed. We favor a Cooper's ligament repair for femoral hernias. In this, we make a relaxing incision into the lower adjacent anterior rectus sheath and bring the free edge of the medial conjoined tendon down to Cooper's ligament, where it is sutured with two or three interrupted sutures. Taking care to avoid injury to the inferior epigastric vessels, a transitional suture is then placed between Cooper's ligament, the femoral sheath, and the conjoined tendon. From there lateralward, the conjoined tendon is sutured to the free shelving border of Poupart's ligament.

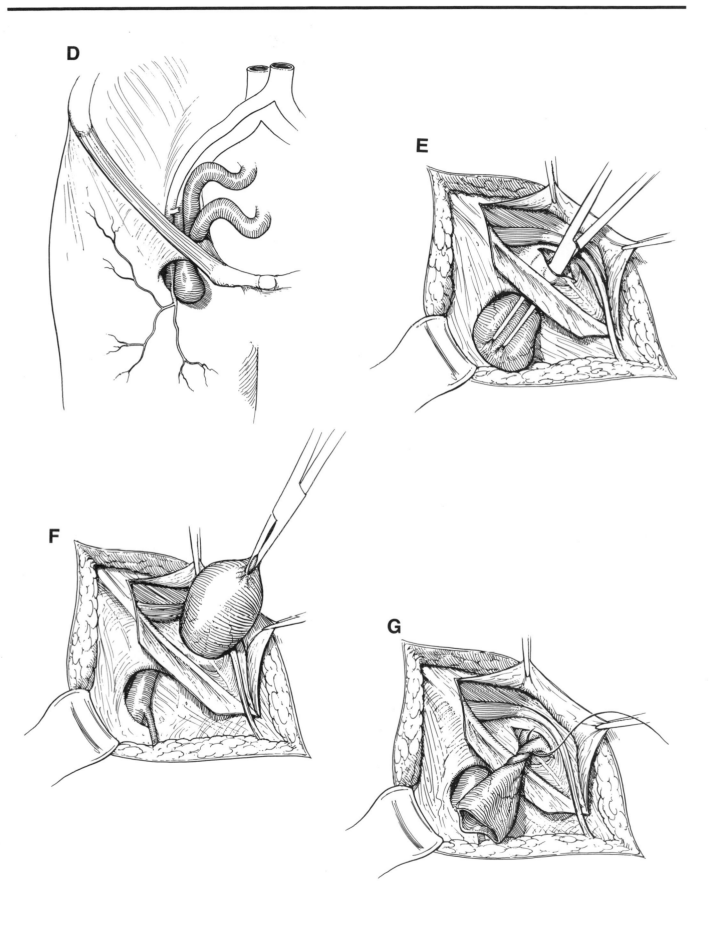

Small Bowel Tumors

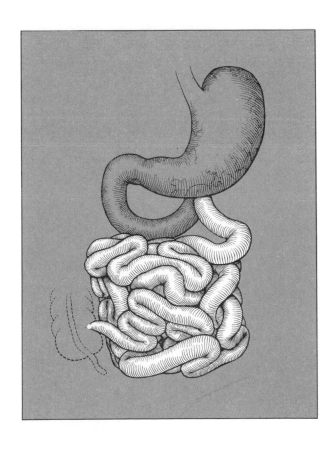

40

Tumors of the small bowel may be benign or malignant. They often are asymptomatic; when symptoms are manifest, they are usually those of either *anemia* or *obstruction* (that is, enteric cramping, diarrhea, distention, and obstipation). Any tumor involving the surface mucosa of the gut will bleed from time to time, and patients may present with symptoms of anemia, as do patients with colonic tumors. Malignant tumors are usually adenocarcinomas, lymphomas, or leiomyosarcomas. Any kind of soft tissue malignancy may involve the small bowel. Benign tumors may be hamartomas, adenomas, hemangiomas, fibromas, lipomas or leiomyomas, among others. Benign tumors can usually be excised locally. Whether or not to excise a complete segment of bowel depends upon whether the tumor can be removed easily without compromising the lumen. Malignant tumors should of course be resected with a good margin (about 10 cm) of normal bowel on each side, along with the subtended wedge of mesentery, so as to remove local and regional lymphatics and lymph nodes.

FIG 40–1

A. Adenocarcinoma of the small bowel is similar to colonic adenocarcinoma. Both often present as apple-core lesions that may cause blood loss and anemia, but after producing constriction of the lumen will cause cramping and intermittent diarrhea and, when the constricted lumen is ultimately plugged by enteric material, obstruction. The material causing the obturator obstruction may later be spontaneously passed, so that intermittent symptoms of obstruction and diarrhea may occur.

B. Malignant soft tissue tumors may appear in any form. This shows a leiomyosarcoma constricting the lumen of the small bowel. The sarcoma rarely may invade the mucosa and bleed.

C. Hamartomas or adenomas may be single or multiple. This shows a solitary adenoma, which was removed locally by enterotomy. Frozen-section biopsy showed no malignancy, so the stalk was oversewn and the enterotomy closed (see Fig 40–2).

D. Benign tumors of the wall of the bowel may grow to sufficient size so as to cause narrowing of the lumen and even obstruction. This tumor could be a fibroma or a lipoma or a leiomyoma. Occasionally, these tumors may become sufficiently large and elongated so as to assume a polypoid shape and may be carried along by peristalsis. At times, they may infarct and bleed. I once operated on a man who had had three severe anemic episodes (one leading to a myocardial infarction) that were ultimately found to be caused by a long polypoid lipoma that was bleeding from its tip.

E. Malignant tumors should be resected with a wide margin of normal bowel and a subtended wedge of mesentery so as to attempt to capture any tumor in lymphatic transit.

F. This figure shows end-to-end anastomosis of the small bowel and repair of the mesentery.

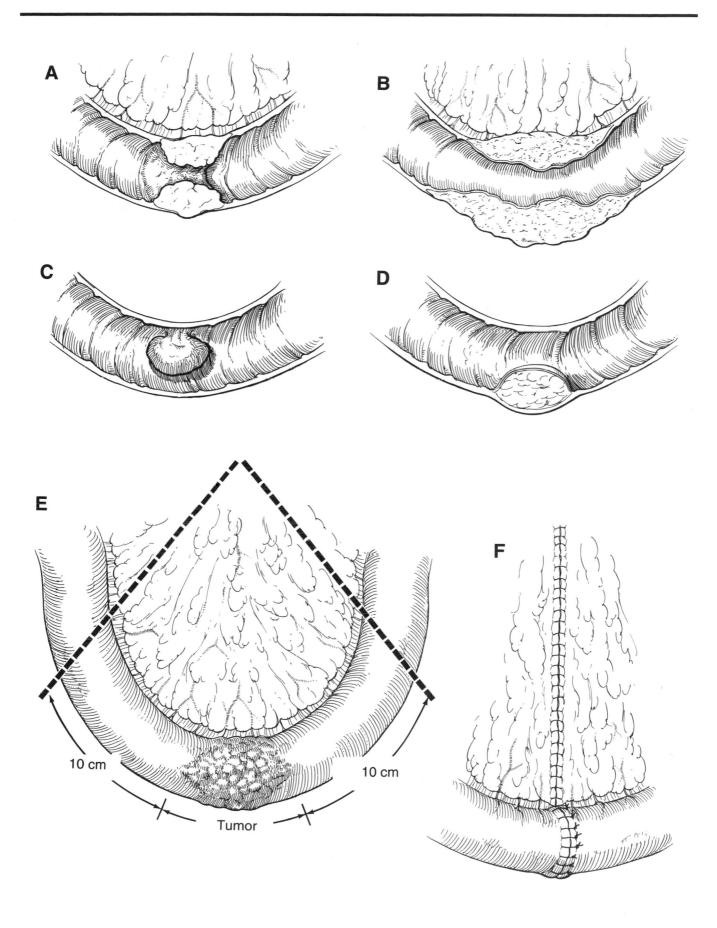

G. The figure depicts transillumination of an area of angiodysplasia in the wall of the small bowel by means of an endoscope within the lumen. Thickness of the vessel wall and the number and area of involved vessels vary. Occasionally the lesion is huge, pulpy, and purple and can easily be visualized on external examination. The illustrated technique of transillumination requires a darkened room and great patience. Since lesions are frequently multiple, demonstration of one area of angiodysplasia calls attention to the possibility that there may be several other areas.

H. Occasionally small bowel intramural tumors may similarly be visualized by transillumination from a light source within the lumen of the bowel. Usually these tumors are palpable but occasionally they are soft and without definite margins and transillumination may be the best way of showing them. Again, the lesions may be multiple so that the entire bowel must be examined.

G

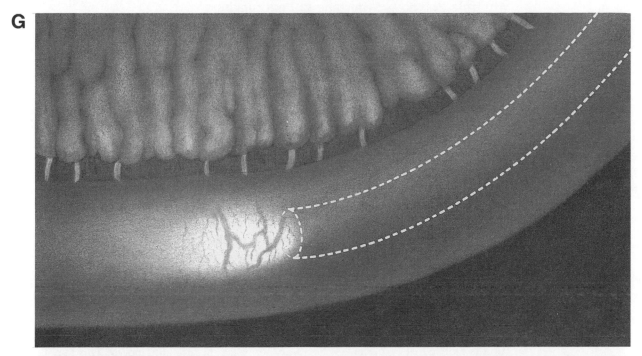

H

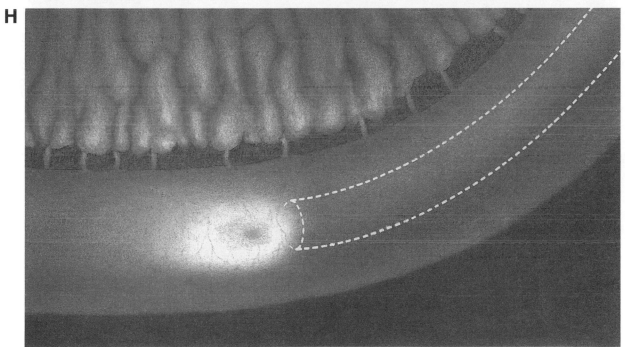

Multiple Polyposis Syndrome of Peutz-Jeghers

The Peutz-Jeghers syndrome consists of multiple hamartomas of the bowel (most often of the small intestine, but any zone of the bowel is susceptible) that give rise to syndromes of hemorrhage or intermittent small bowel obstruction (especially intermittent obstructive episodes that resolve spontaneously). The syndrome is also characterized by melanin spots in the buccal mucosa, usually under the tongue and around the lips and in the fingers, and frequently in the interdigital webs. Any patient who has a history of intermittent episodes of bowel obstruction that resolve spontaneously should be suspected of the Peutz-Jeghers syndrome, especially if the patient demonstrates the melanin stigmata.

FIG 40—2

A. This shows a bleeding hamartomatous polyp that has also initiated intussusception. The bleeding is usually intermittent and may be localized by isotopic scans. Patients may have hundreds of polyps and it is vital, of course, to find the polyp that is bleeding. Localization may require interoperative endoscopy, either through the mouth or through a gastrotomy or enterotomy. Excision of all polyps is usually impractical, so that it is important to find the offending one. Malignancy has been reported but it must be rare.

B. Intussusception gives rise to classic symptoms of small bowel obstruction and, if unrelieved, may of course lead to necrosis of the intussuscepted segment. At operation, it may be possible easily to relieve the intussusception, but usually there is sufficient swelling so that the reduction is difficult, if not impossible, and the whole area should be resected. If intussusception is reduced, it is, of course, necessary to excise the offending polyp. This may be accomplished by putting an endoscope in at some distance and removing the polyp endoscopically, thereby avoiding an enterotomy in edematous bowel.

C. Commonly, the Peutz-Jeghers polyp that leads the intussusception may infarct and fall off and the intussusception may reduce itself spontaneously. This is actually fairly common and many patients will give long histories of intermittent episodes of cramping abdominal pain, abdominal distention, nausea, and vomiting that disappear spontaneously.

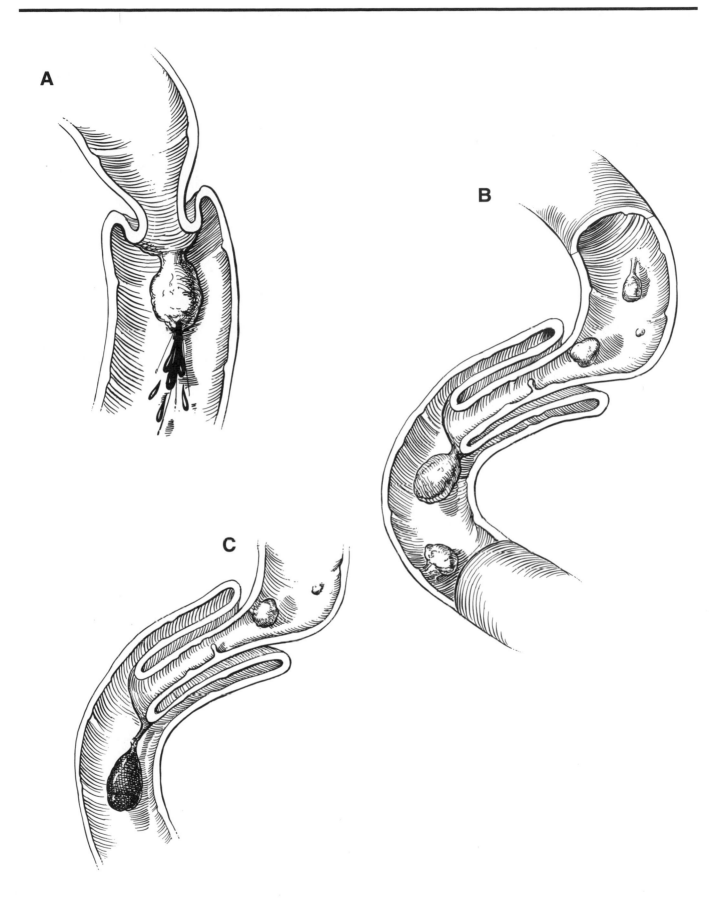

Crohn's Disease
of the Small Bowel

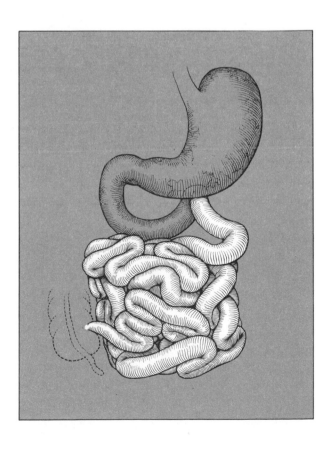

41

Crohn's disease is the most common surgical disease of the small intestine. Given this, it is surprising to consider that the disease entity was unknown until described with almost blinding accuracy by Crohn, Ginzburg, and Oppenheimer in 1932 (*JAMA* 1932; 99:1323). They did err initially in assuming that the process was confined to the terminal ileum. We now know that the condition, whose pathologic features are well recognized but whose etiology and pathogenesis are, as yet, unraveled, can affect any part of the gut from the esophagus to the anus. The small bowel is involved in 85% of patients (more than half of all patients with Crohn's disease have involvement of the ileum and colon). The incidence of Crohn's disease seems to be influenced by geography and by economics. The disease is most common in North America and Northern Europe and it is becoming more common; some epidemiologic evidence suggests that the incidence doubled from 1963 to 1973 in the United States. Within a community, hospitals with a relatively affluent clientele will see far more patients with Crohn's disease than will be seen in institutions with indigent patients. Pathologic changes are characterized by edema, hyperemia, stenosing lymphangitis, mucosal ulceration, and thickening of the bowel wall (which becomes shortened and rigid). At operation, the surgeon sees thickened loops of bowel with short, thick mesentery. Areas of diseased bowel are often separated by grossly normal bowel, so-called "skip areas." Extensive fat-wrapping, caused by circumferential growth of mesenteric fat around the external wall of the bowel, is a striking finding of Crohn's disease. The bowel wall is thick, firm, rubbery, incompressible. Proximal uninvolved bowel is often dilated because of stenosis of the diseased segments. Often multiple loops will be matted together into a conglomerate mass, often containing internal fistulas. Mesenteric nodes may be massively enlarged and succulent. Single areas of involvement are more common than multiple, and the distal ileum is the most common site of the disease. Clinical manifestations often begin in young adults with recurring and persistent abdominal pain, usually cramping, diarrhea, weight loss, and fever. Perianal fistula disease is common; it is found in one out of four patients with small bowel Crohn's disease. Any patient with chronic recurring episodes of abdominal pain, especially those of long duration, diarrhea, and weight loss should be suspected of having Crohn's disease, as should any patient with multiple perineal fecal fistulas. The diagnosis is usually made by barium study of the small bowel, and many authorities suggest that radiographic enteroclysis is probably the best study. Surprisingly, there is little correlation between the degree of radiographic severity and clinical manifestations of the disease, so that radiographic studies should be prompted by symptoms and not just by previous radiographic studies. There is no cure for Crohn's disease. Medical treatment is largely symptomatic and empiric. Surgical treatment is directed towards correction of specific complications (obstruction, abscess, symptomatic fistulas, free perforation, ureteral obstruction, bleeding, cancer, or failure to thrive). At operation, resection should be limited to the segment of bowel responsible for the complication that precipitated operations, even if adjacent (and distant) areas are clearly diseased. Asymptomatic fistulas are not an indication for operation. Management of symptomatic fistulas should be direct and as simple as possible. If the fistula is between two diseased loops of bowel, diseased segments of both loops should be excised and anastomosed. If, however, the fistula is between a diseased loop of small bowel and an apparently normal area of small intestine or colon or bladder, the diseased loop of small bowel should be excised and anastomosed, the fistula orifice should be simply excised from the wall of the normal structure, and the opening in the normal structure should be simply closed. Free perforation is uncommon; when present it usually occurs in a diseased segment of bowel, but may also occur in relatively normal bowel proximal to obstruction. The perforated segment should be resected back to grossly relatively normal bowel on each side and anastomosed. At no time should the surgeon attempt to eradicate the disease. There is no place for frozen section biopsy of the line of resection, since there is no therapeutic justification for excision of all apparently diseased bowel. At operation, we are after only segments that obstruct or perforate or bleed. When the focal point of the operation is in the terminal ileum, the distal line of resection should be in the ascending colon, and no attempt should be made to do a standard right colectomy, although it is technically easier. There should be no effort to remove enlarged lymph nodes, since their excision does not alter recurrence and may interfere with blood supply of the bowel. Likewise, previously popular bypass procedures with exclusion should be limited only to elderly patients who are poor surgical risks or patients with multiple prior resections and very short bowel, and in patients in whom resection would require entering an abscess or causing danger to some normal structure. In recent years, several surgeons have attempted to avoid resection of strictured zones of small intestine by utilizing a local procedure, strictureplasty, as an alternative to resection. This is a variation of the Heineke-Milkulicz procedure, in which there is longitudinal incision of the stricture, including about 1 cm of bowel on either side, with transverse closure of the incision. Enthusiasts for the method say that there is no increased incidence of leaks or recurrence as compared to resection. We do not use the method. We do not believe that anyone should be confused: the standard treatment of obstructing or bleeding or fistulous segments of Crohn's disease is limited resection and anastomosis of the diseased bowel. Cancer is not a common complication of Crohn's disease of the small intestine, but it is said to be 100 times more common in patients with Crohn's disease of the ileum, for example, than in normal individuals of the same age. Crohn's disease does tend to burn out and active disease is unusual after 55 years, but it does occur. Townsend and I have discussed Crohn's disease in the fifth edition of Schwartz's *Principles of Surgery* (New York, McGraw-Hill, 1969, pp 1198–1202). I will illustrate several different areas of involvement and how they might be managed at operation.

FIG 41 – 1

A. A short area of profound Crohn's ileitis producing partial obstruction (not involving the ileum immediately adjacent to the ileocecal valve) should be treated by local resection.

B. The area of excision should be confined to the most severely diseased portion and no attempt should be made to dissect out lymph nodes up to the origin of the ileocolic artery.

C. After the grossly abnormal bowel is excised, the remaining ileum is anastomosed and the rent in the mesentery repaired.

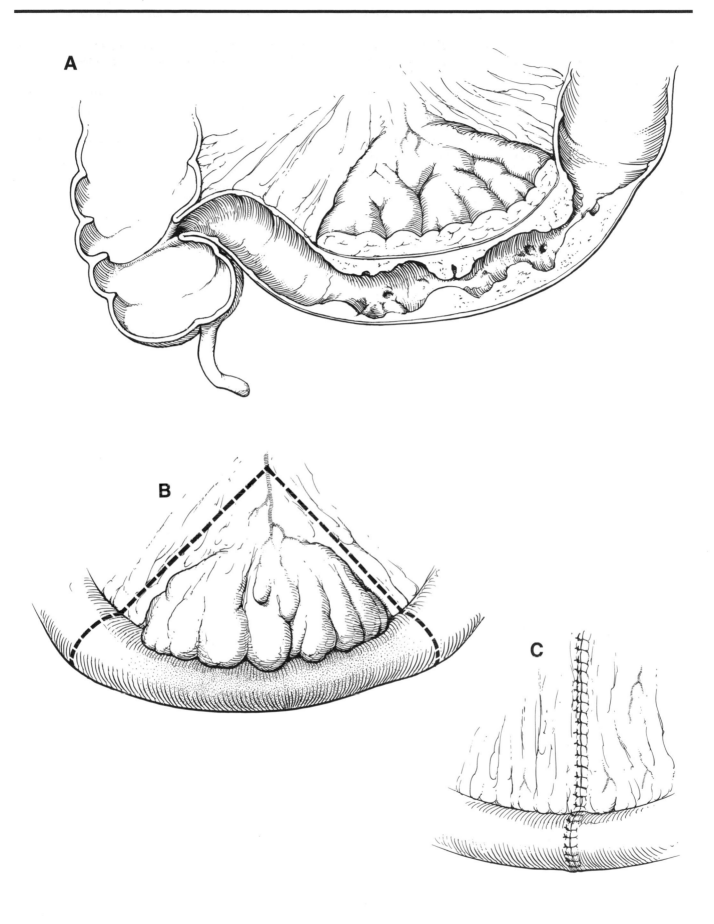

D. Enterocutaneous fistulas should be managed by excising the area of grossly involved small intestine and debriding the fistulous tract through the abdominal wall from the inside.

E. After the bowel is reanastomosed, it should be separated, if at all possible, from the abdominal wall with omental fat. A small drain should be placed temporarily in the tract of the abdominal wall fistula.

F. When an enteroenteric fistula connects a loop of badly diseased bowel with a loop of relatively normal bowel, the abnormal segment of bowel should be excised and the bowel reanastomosed, whereas the fistulous opening into the loop of normal bowel should be simply excised and closed locally.

G. When two grossly abnormal segments of bowel have a short intervening segment of apparently normal bowel, the question arises as to whether or not to try to save the normal "skip area" (shown in detail in Figs **H–K,** p. 313).

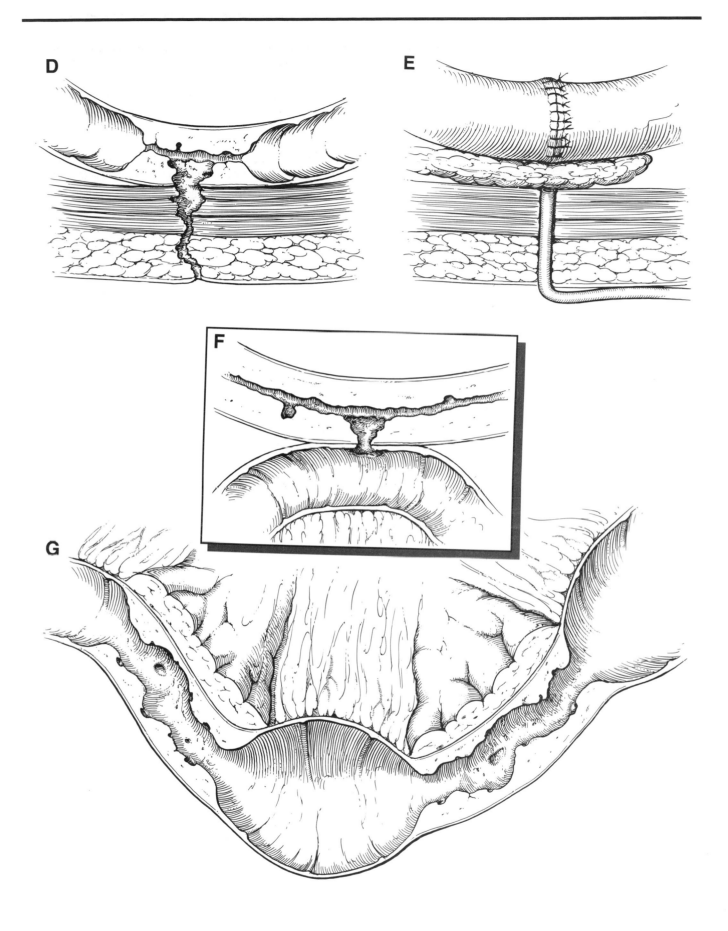

H. The answer depends upon the length of the intervening normal segment. If it is 10 cm or greater, it probably should be saved. If it is 5 cm or less, it should be taken.

I. Both areas would be excised in this instance, but each case must be individualized, and the answer will depend also upon the configuration of the blood supply, the mobility of the mesentery, and other local factors. If previous resections have left the bowel critically short, we may go to great lengths to preserve small segments.

J. When the terminal ileum and ascending colon are involved in a confluent process, a formal right colectomy is indicated providing that the ascending colon is so diseased that connecting the ileum to it would be hazardous.

K. If there are one or more additional areas of uncomplicated Crohn's disease *(arrows),* these should be left alone.

L. When an involved loop of bowel perforates locally into the mesentery, creating an adjacent abscess, the involved segment of bowel and the entire intramesenteric abscess should be excised, taking care, if possible, to remove the mass without opening the abscess.

Small Bowel

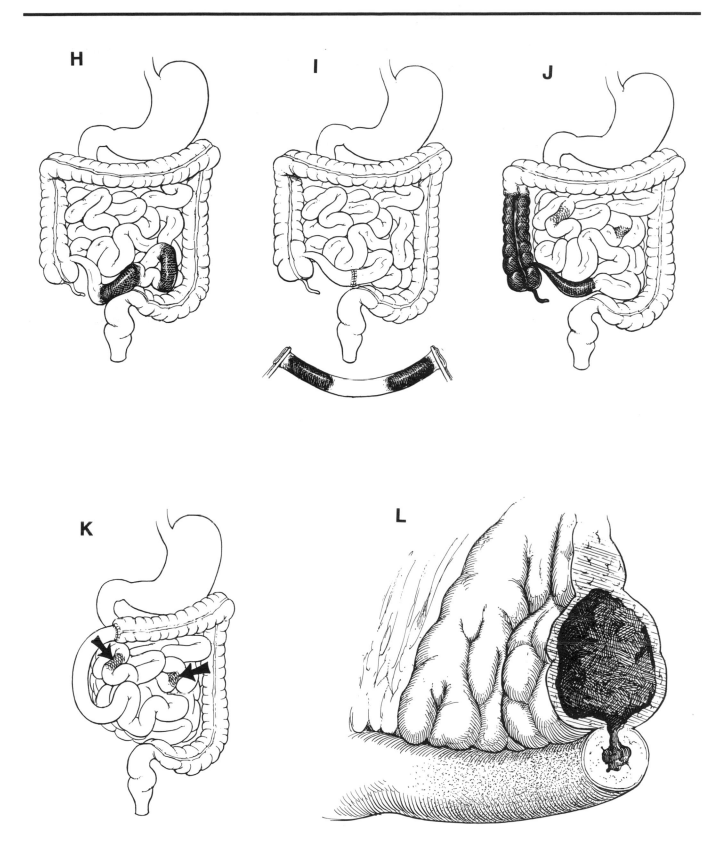

M. The extent of surgical resection in patients with Crohn's disease depends upon the extent of critical involvement. This complex lesion includes an enterocolic and enterovesical fistula, with involvement of a relatively large segment of the wall of the sigmoid and a small segment of the bladder wall. This lesion was treated by excisions as indicated here by dotted *lines*. We decided to excise the short colon segment because of the large zone of fusion between ileum and colon, and because of the large area of colonic induration.

N. The resected specimen includes the limb of ileum with adjacent involved loop of sigmoid and a rim of bladder.

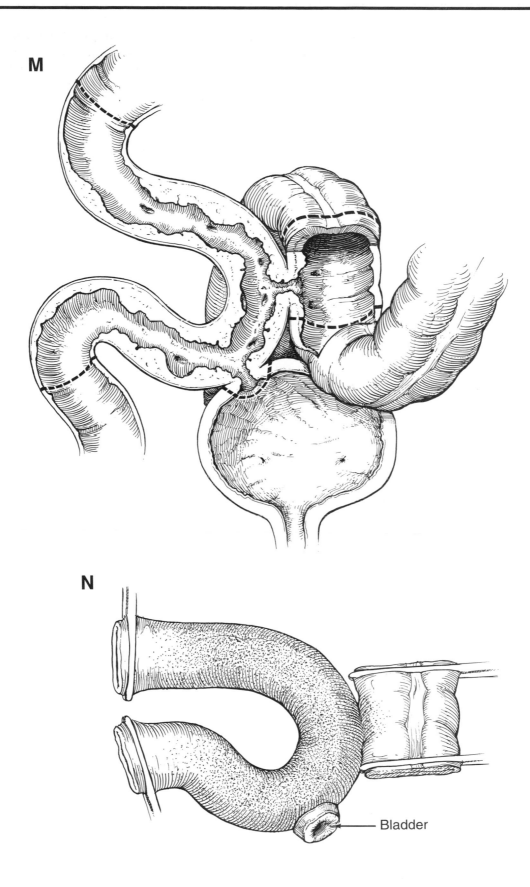

Bladder

O. This shows the anastomosed ileum and sigmoid and the repaired bladder with indwelling catheter. No attempt is made to eradicate disease; only those areas that cause serious threats are excised.

O

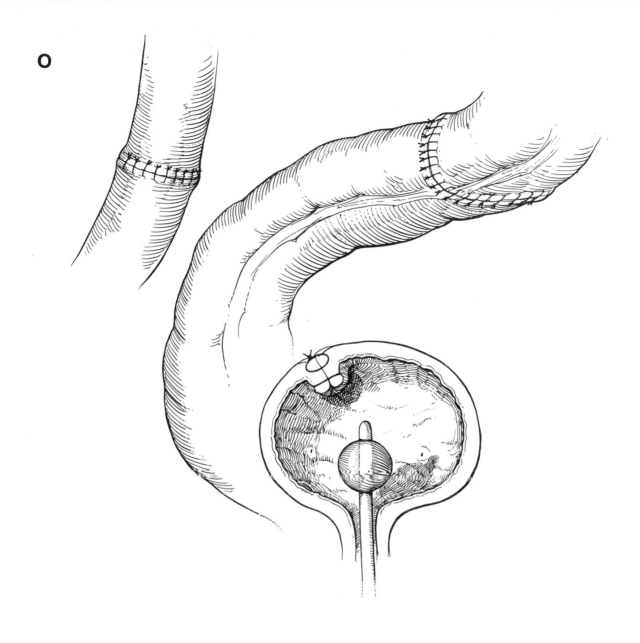

Techniques

42

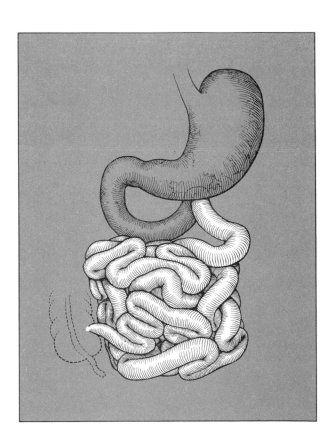

End-to-End Sutured Anastomosis of the Small Bowel

The time may well come when bowel anastomoses are all done by machines, but until that time, the ability to safely construct hand-sewn bowel anastomoses is a cornerstone of abdominal surgery. The main requisite for success is good blood supply of the bowel to be anastomosed. Care should be taken to avoid tension, to provide an adequate lumen, and if possible, to avoid blind loops or cul-de-sacs of bowel. I routinely use a two-layer anastomosis, although I know many good surgeons who use a single layer.

FIG 42–1

A. I use 4-0 polyglactin (Vicryl) sutures on small Ferguson needles, although I recognize now that most surgeons use swaged-on sutures. Many surgeons observe that in a two-layer anastomosis, there are often more serosal sutures on the anterior row than on the posterior. The reason is that the anterior row, once the clamps are taken off, constitutes more than 50% of the circumference of the bowel (that is, the bowel balloons open once unclamped).

B. The through-and-through posterior row of sutures is applied with 3-0 or 4-0 swaged polyglactin sutures placed adjacent to one another on the posterior row and then tied together. Each is then sewn in opposite directions in a running, locking fashion to complete the posterior row, and then brought around anteriorly as a Connell stitch. Obvious generalizations about sutures are that the closer to the wound margin the stitch is taken, the more sutures needed, and secondly, the fewer sutures taken, the more tissue turned in. We take time to clamp and ligate any small bleeders that persist after removal of the clamps. We put mosquito clamps on these vessels and place only two knots on the ties, and do this quickly, but the attention has prevented troublesome postoperative suture-line bleeding.

C. The anastomosis is completed with an anterior row of interrupted 4-0 polyglactin sutures. Confirmation of a patent lumen can be made by placing the thumb and forefingers through the anastomotic lumen, invaginating full thickness of bowel on each side.

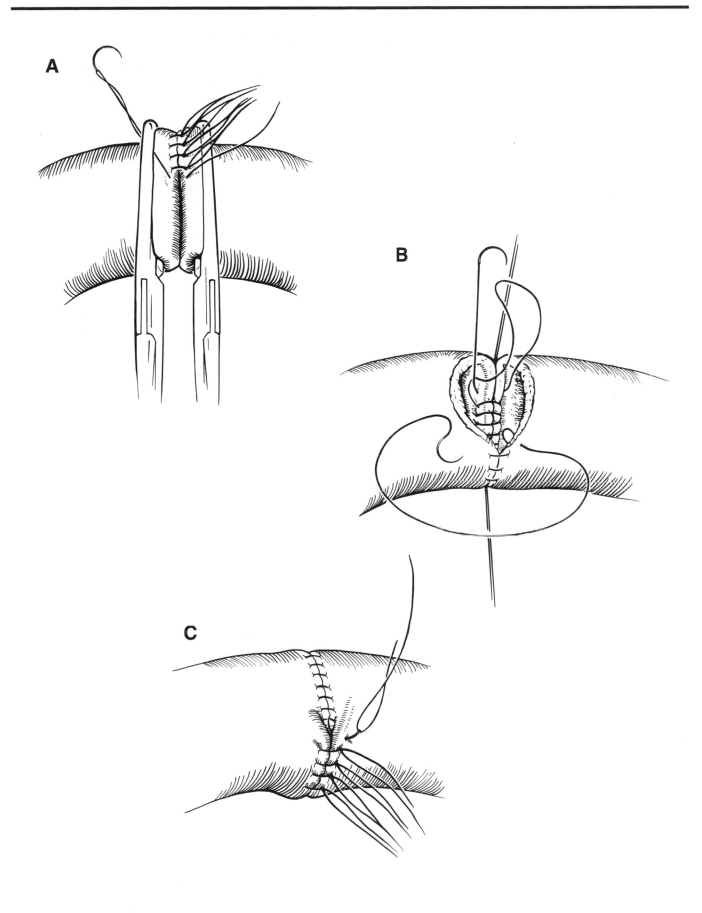

Operative Placement of an Enterostomy Tube (Witzel Technique)

Small catheter enterostomies placed through a needle are often unsatisfactory: they leak, they become occluded, and they are of insufficient diameter to allow efficient suction. A large plastic catheter (12 to 14 F) can be safely placed by creating a serosal tunnel to shield the enterostomy site. This so-called Witzel technique allows placement of tubes for instillation of enteric feedings or for decompression.

FIG 42–2

A. A site is selected on the antimesenteric border of the small bowel, a pursestring 4-0 suture is placed, and an enterotomy is created inside the suture ring.

B. The enterostomy tube is inserted to the desired length and the pursestring suture ligated.

C. A row of interrupted serosal 4-0 sutures is then placed in such a manner as to duck the tube and create a serosal tunnel. Here we have placed two sutures distal to the enterotomy and eight sutures proximal.

D. This shows the completed enterostomy tube placement. The insert shows a cross section of the enterostomy tube in the serosal tunnel. We usually bring out the tube through a stab wound in the abdominal wall and fix the tube by polyglactin suture to the internal and external surfaces of the abdominal wall.

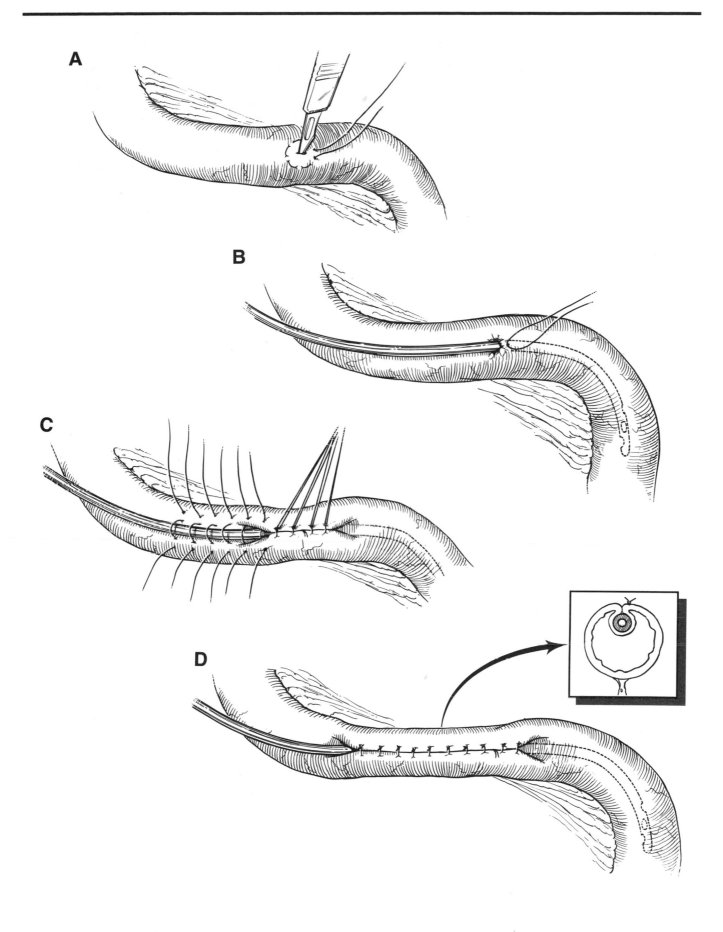

Ileostomy (Brooke)

Meticulous technique is essential in formation of a well-functioning ileostomy. Ileostomy dysfunction is common and ileal stomas frequently require revision. Most surgeons have adopted the technique of Brooke, which includes suturing the mucosa to the skin margin (so-called early maturation) so as to afford an early seal and thereby minimize the complications of serositis, subcutaneous abscesses, and intramural perforation of the ileum. Stomal therapists have great experience with the management of both happy and cranky ileostomies. We always seek their counsel in the placement of the ileostomy and we depend on their help for familiarizing the patient with postoperative care of the ileal stoma. Other patients with well-functioning ileostomies are often a great help to an individual contemplating having an ileostomy. They will familiarize the patient with the best way successfully to cope with the ileostomy. Some ileostomies put out huge quantities of fluid in the first several days after operation, but the volume is usually down to 200 to 300 mL within 2 to 4 weeks. Many recent modifications have threatened to render the ileostomy either obsolete (mucosal proctectomy and ileoanal anastomosis), or continent (the Koch ileostomy or the Mayo Clinic intraluminal balloon-plug ileostomy appliance), but since the dust hasn't yet settled, discussion will be limited here to the formation of a simple Brooke ileostomy.

FIG 42–3

A. Selection of the site is the first important decision and should be made before operation. Stomal therapists often recommend an exact spot that will allow convenient placement of the foreplate of an ileostomy bag. If the placement is too low or too lateral, it may be difficult to achieve a good seal, and this may lead to later serious problems. After careful selection, the site is marked with indelible ink. At operation the skin is picked up with an Allis clamp and a disk of skin excised. The disk should be about the size of a dime or slightly larger (a diameter of 1.8 to 2.0 cm). The excision is initiated as shown, but as soon as the skin is incised, the line of incision through the skin should be vertical, so as to have a full-thickness plug of skin, with no beveled edges.

B. After hemostasis is secure in the subcutaneous tissue, the rectus fascia overlying the lower right rectus muscle is incised and a clamp placed through the muscle and into the peritoneal cavity. It is important to have the aperture just the right size. Too small and the ileostomy function will be impeded by stenosis; too large and the ileostomy is apt to prolapse. The surgeon should place a finger through the wound to gauge the opening in the rectus fascia; if the fascia seems to have a sharp edge causing pressure on the examining finger, the opening should be dilated or the sharp edge excised locally. After the aperture has been fully developed, a clamp is placed through the opening to grasp the ileal stoma. We place the clamp immediately behind the occluding clamp held within the abdomen, remove the intra-abdominal clamp, and pull the ileum through the anterior abdominal wall. If the size of the aperture is correct, it will be possible to do this, but the fit will be tight.

C. The protruding ileal segment should be about 5 cm long. The crushed tip is cut off with a knife and hemostasis carefully secured.

D. We placed a series of 4-0 polyglactin (Vicryl) sutures through the full thickness of the ileostomy and through the full thickness of the skin so that it will be possible to evert the mucosa and sew it down to the skin.

E. The completed everted stoma should protrude 2 to 3 cm from the surface. The folding back of mucosa (so-called maturation) protects against inflammation and gives the protruding ileal nipple a thicker wall and more substance.

F. Within the abdomen, the serosa of the bowel should be sewn circumferentially to the peritoneum to prevent prolapse. We tack the ileal mesentery to the peritoneum of the anterior body wall and then to the lateral body wall, so as to mitigate against twisting of the small bowel around the fixed ileostomy.

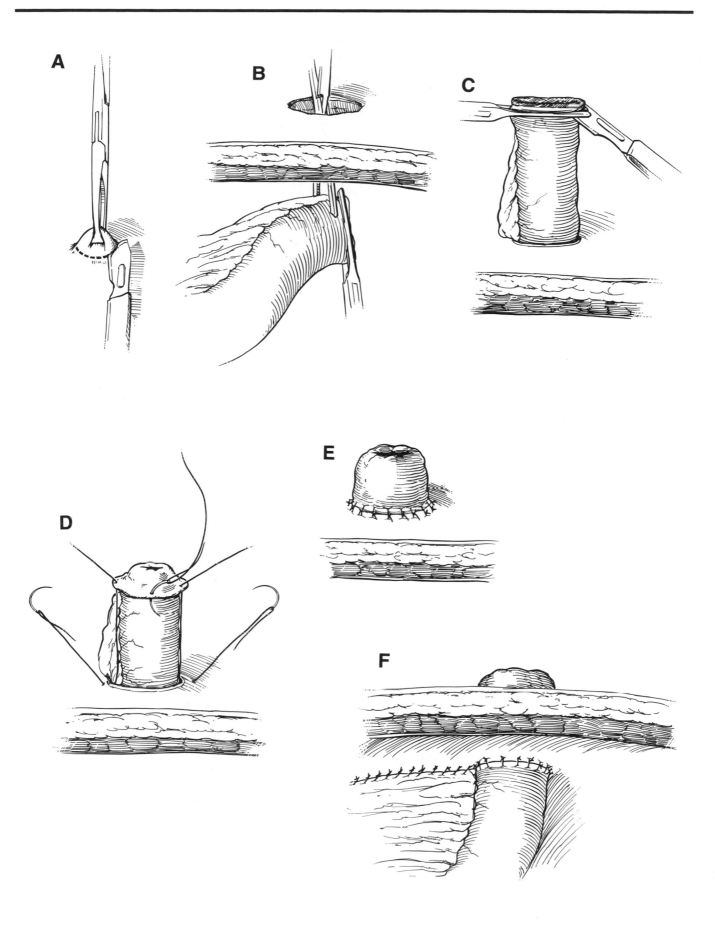

Drainage of Pancreatic Pseudocyst Cystogastrostomy or Roux-en-Y Cystojejunostomy

Development of ultrasonographic methods for demonstrating intra-abdominal pathology has greatly improved our ability to deal with pancreatic pseudocysts. Although we always understood that some cysts went away spontaneously, we had scant criteria for predicting which ones would require operative treatment. Indications for operation in patients with pancreatic pseudocysts are those of gut dysfunction (usually gastric or duodenal obstruction) or, rarely, hemorrhage. Since we are dealing here with surgery of the stomach, duodenum, and small bowel, we will limit discussion to relief of obstructive symptoms. It is, however, worth noting that in patients with large bleeding pseudocysts, a transthoracic approach through the sixth interspace, opening the diaphragm and approaching the pseudocyst from above and behind, often allows direct ligation of the splenic artery by way of an approach that is much simpler than wading through bloody pseudocyst contents in a transcystic approach. Similarly, it is not possible to evaluate here the relative indications for percutaneous drainage, other than to say that many skilled interventional radiologists have been successful in draining pseudocysts by percutaneous catheterization. We have seen many of their failures (owing to clogging of the tubes by thick intracystic debris), and some surgeons have developed a prejudice against percutaneous drainage. It certainly does work in many relatively simple cysts and is a simple solution in what might otherwise be a case that required operation. Another difficult decision is whether infected pseudocysts should be marsupialized (that is, drained externally), or drained into the gut. Despite published warnings by some students of the disease that all infected pseudocysts should be drained externally, we drain most of them into the gut. If the patient has an obvious abscess in a pseudocyst, we drain it externally. But if the patient has a few WBCs and bacteria in the cyst fluid, we perform internal drainage; such drainage will work unless contamination is severe. In performing intraoperative drainage, the site of anastomosis of the cyst depends upon the location of the cyst. If the cyst is tightly applied to the posterior wall of the stomach, it is best drained into the stomach. For some reason, this procedure works. A priori, one might consider that gastric contents would empty into the cyst, digest the cyst, and wreak havoc, but that usually doesn't happen, and cystgastrostomy is the most common method of internal drainage. If the cyst impinges on the wall of the duodenum, an anastomosis can be made between the cyst and the duodenum. If the cyst is not tightly applied to the wall of any part of the gut, it is probably best to create a Roux-en-Y segment of jejunum and perform a direct anastomosis between the Roux limb and the cyst.

FIG 42–4

A. This upper GI series shows pressure on and lateral displacement of the distal stomach by a pseudocyst of the body of the pancreas. The *arrows* show the proximal margin of cyst pressure, which effaces the mucosal pattern. The cyst greatly impedes emptying of the stomach. At operation, the cyst was found to be tightly applied to the posterior wall of the stomach, and a highly effective cystogastrostomy was performed.

B. Ultrasonography is probably the best diagnostic study in patients with pancreatic pseudocysts. One of the great advantages of ultrasonography is that it allows an appreciation of the thickness of the wall and of the homogeneity (or lack of it) of the cyst contents, and often tells us whether the cyst is multilocular. This cross-sectional ultrasonogram shows a large pancreatic pseudocyst, the walls of which are thin (as noted by the *arrows*). Cyst wall thickness is thought by many to be a gauge of the "maturity" of the cyst. Thin-walled cysts often resolve spontaneously; thick-walled cysts do so rarely. The spine in this figure is indicated by an *s* and the kidney by a *k*.

C. This cross-sectional ultrasonogram depicts a thick-walled pancreatic pseudocyst (thickness of wall denoted by *arrows*). At operation this thick-walled cyst was drained into the stomach.

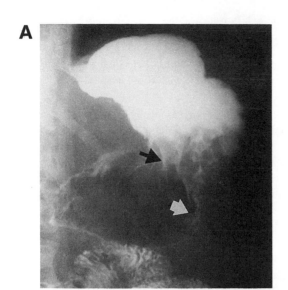

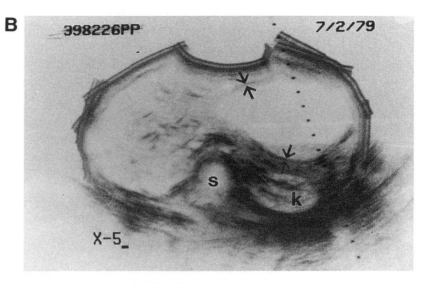

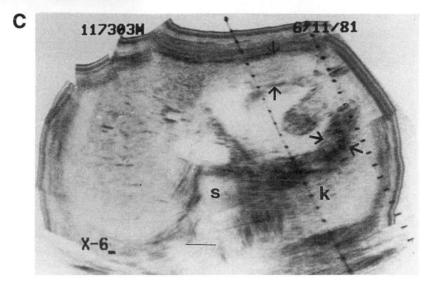

D. This figure diagrammatically illustrates the relationship of the stomach, pancreas, and a retrogastric pseudocyst of the body of the pancreas.

E. This cross-sectional diagram shows the cyst lying between the stomach and pancreas exerting pressure on the posterior gastric wall.

F. After an anterior gastrotomy is made along the dotted line shown in **D,** hemostasis is secured and the retrogastric mass palpated through the posterior wall of the stomach. The surgeon should perform needle aspiration of this mass bulging into the posterior wall in order to be sure that an incision through the posterior gastric wall will, in fact, go into the pseudocyst. If, as anticipated, the aspirate shows cloudy, grumous, dark fluid typical of a pseudocyst, we proceded with cystogastrostomy. If the aspirate is pure pus, we will likely close the gastrotomy, open up the abscess through the gastrocolonic ligament, clean out all pus and debris, and drain it. If we had anticipated dealing with an abscess, we would not have opened the stomach.

G. We next cut out an ellipse of fused posterior gastric wall and anterior wall of the cyst with the electrocautery. As soon as the cyst is entered, there will be a flow of grumous fluid. This should be aspirated, and if it appears to be infected, we will obtain Gram stain and aerobic and anaerobic cultures.

H. The entire cyst should be visualized. A lighted retractor is often helpful.

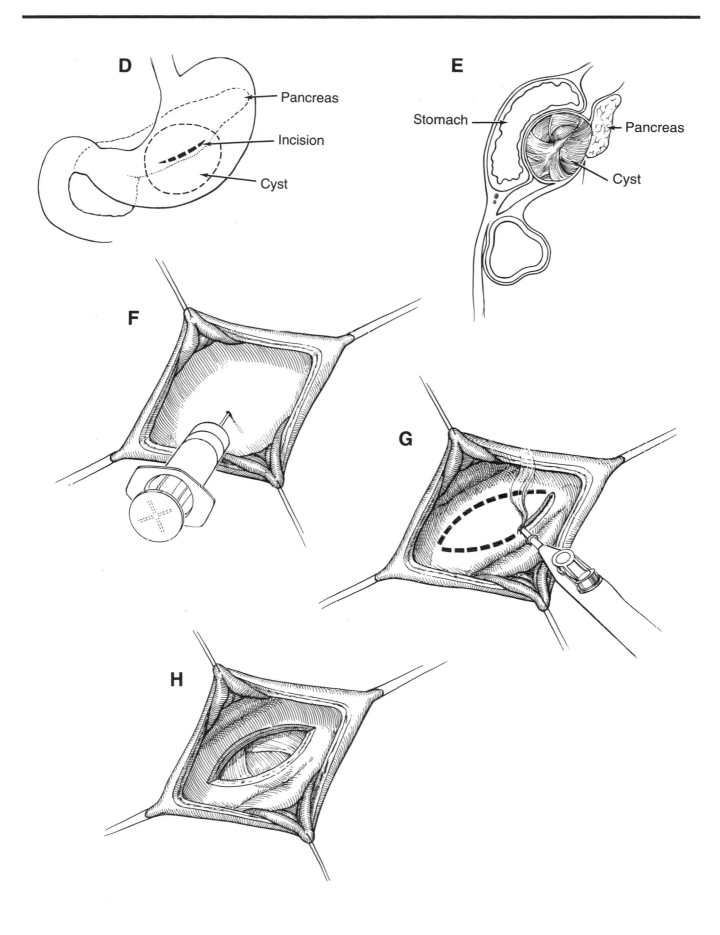

I. The cyst should be carefully inspected. Cysts are often multilocular, and loculations must be broken down so as to allow complete drainage of the cyst. If the loculations are thick, we would prefer to remove them by electrocautery rather than by finger dissection, as shown here.

J. We usually run a continuous locking suture around the wall of the cystogastrostomy so as to achieve hemostasis and to mitigate against spontaneous closure of the opening. Some surgeons have spoken against this step, suggesting that it facilitates drainage of gastric juice into the cyst and digestion of the cyst wall, but we have not had that complication, and we are secure in doing this in order to prevent reformation of the cyst.

K. The anterior gastrotomy is then closed with two Connell through-and-through running sutures, reinforced with a row of interrupted 4-0 polyglactin sutures.

L. The cyst usually collapses completely and results are usually good. Occasionally we have had bleeding from the wall of the cystogastrostomy, even with the running locking suture. On the two occasions in which this happened, we were able to stop the bleeding by cauterization by means of gastroscopy.

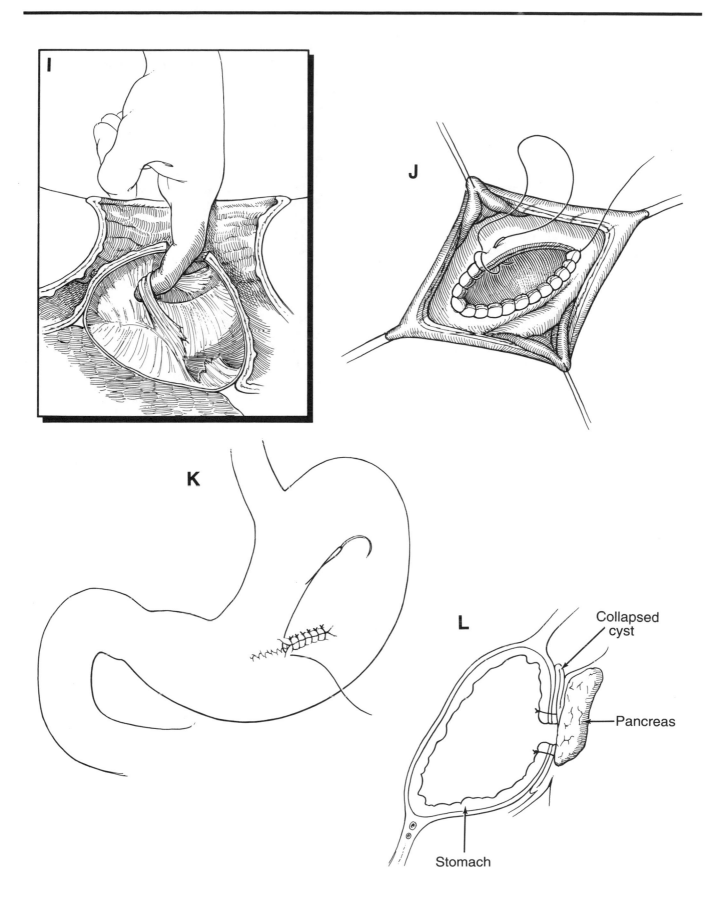

I

J

K

L

Collapsed
cyst

Pancreas

Stomach

M. This is a sagittal view showing a multilocular pancreatic pseudocyst pressing on the posterior wall of the stomach, the transverse mesocolon, and the transverse colon.

N. This is an anterior view showing the pseudocyst pressing on the greater curvature of the stomach and on the splenic flexure of the colon. Occasionally, the pseudocyst has no contact at all with the stomach and is best drained by a Roux-en-Y pancreatic cystojejunostomy.

O. The principle of enteric drainage is the same whether it is performed into the stomach or into an isolated limb of jejunum. When using the jejunum, the Roux-en-Y limb is mobilized by dividing the proximal jejunum about 12 to 15 cm distal to the ligament of Treitz. We select the exact point of division by visualizing the vascular arcade in the jejunal mesentery and dividing it at a point that will ensure good blood supply. The jejunum is divided, as shown here, with the GIA stapling device.

P. The Roux-en-Y limb is brought superiorly through an opening in the transverse mesocolon into approximation with the pseudocyst.

Q. A routine two-layer anastomosis is performed between the cyst and the jejunum. First, a posterior row of interrupted sutures is placed so as to provide for an anastomosis closely adjacent to the stapled end of the jejunum. Openings are then made in adjacent walls of the cyst and the jejunum and hemostasis is secured. The cyst is explored (as shown in **I**) in order to break down any possible loculations. A posterior running suture of swaged 3-0 polyglactin is then placed to go full-thickness through the walls of the cyst and the jejunum. This suture is then brought around anteriorly in a continuous inverting Connell suture. The anterior suture line is then reinforced within interrupted polyglactin sutures.

R. This figure shows the finished pancreatic cystojejunostomy Roux-en-Y. A jejunojejunostomy is then performed to reestablish continuity of the gut (see Chapter 25).

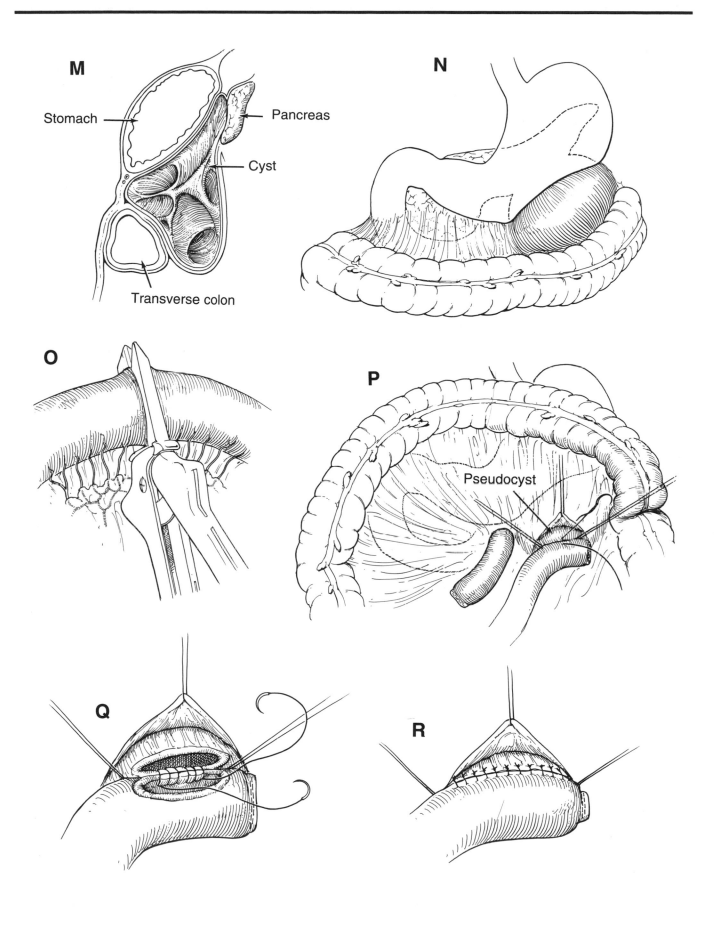

M

Stomach

Pancreas

Cyst

Transverse colon

N

O

P

Pseudocyst

Q

R

Index